MW00352400

By Charles Moore

The Black Market: a guide to art collecting

Israel's Transformative Black Artists

The Brilliance of the Color Black Through the Eyes of Art Collectors

APROPOS OF RUNNING

Apropos of
Running

A memoir

Charles Moore

Petite ✦ Ivy
PRESS

Apropos of Running: a memoir NEW YORK, NEW YORK, U.S.A.

Copyright ©2023 by CHARLES MOORE.
All rights reserved.
Published in the United States by Petite Ivy Press.
All images, logos, quotes, and trademarks included in this book are subject to use according to trademark and copyright laws of the United States of America.
Library of Congress Control Number:
Names: MOORE, CHARLES, Author
Title: Apropos of Running: a memoir / CHARLES MOORE
Description: New York: Petite Ivy Press. [2023]
Identifiers: LCCN 2023945155 (print) |
ISBN: 978-1-955496-08-7 (hardcover print) | ISBN: 978-1-955496-13-1 (ebook)

QUANTITY PURCHASES: Schools, companies, professional groups, clubs, and other organizations may qualify for special terms when ordering quantities of this title.

Portrait painter: Telvin Wallace

Cover Design: David Jon Walker

For Columbus Jr., Cheryl & Andrea

Table of Contents

Chapter 01
"Be"

At the Detroit Free Press Marathon, when I finally arrived at the starting line, I felt relieved and accomplished—mainly because I'd be running in front of a home crowd. I'm originally from the Motor City, a place that helped shape some of my greatest hopes and dreams.

Because this race crosses into Canada, it is considered an international race, which comes with all sorts of terrorism threats. There are specific rules in place for Detroit, not to be broken. First, anyone not running is not allowed on the course. Second, runners must show their bibs at all times.

My engine started revving up around mile twelve; my stride was unbroken while racing up Bagley Street. Just then, I spotted two Black police officers, and one motioned for me to unzip my jacket. *I'm freezing,* I thought as I reluctantly followed orders. My engine was just taking off, so compliance didn't seem like too big a deal.

As I passed the two Black officers, a White officer was just behind them. He jumped off his post and placed his left arm out as his right hand went for his pistol.

Is this guy seriously going for his gun? I wondered. *I am a Black man from Detroit; maybe this is business as usual for this guy. Sad.*

When I had first started running races, I had just turned forty. Being newly "over the hill," I set three goals for myself as a runner and as a Black man: to inspire the next generation of Black youth, including my nieces and nephews; to challenge myself to new heights as a human and prove to myself and others than I was enough; and to create a community for myself. Up to this point, with about a dozen marathons and races under my belt, I wasn't sure I had achieved any of my initial goals. And now I wasn't sure I was going to finish this race, much less make it out alive.

"I need to see your bib!" the officer shouted.

"You can talk to me, but don't you dare put your hands on me, or by the time I'm done suing you, I'll be renting your home out for extra income," I blurted out in frustration.

Wait. What did I just do? Should I stop for this man or keep running? I don't think I can outrun him. I need to finish today. I have to win.

^^^

As far back as I can remember, I have always wanted to win at everything. My mother, Cheryl, was very competitive, and since I take after her in many ways, so was I. For her, it mostly came out when we had the family over to play Monopoly, Scrabble, or card games like spades. Mine was scholarly tournaments at school and shooting hoops in the neighborhood. I dreamed of hearing, "Go, Charles!" chanted on the basketball court after a killer crossover move or thunderous cheers when I smoked some unsuspecting kid in an Academic Games League of America (AGLOA) tournament. Now in its fiftieth year, AGLOA consists of local, regional, and national tournaments that test adolescents' abilities in logic, mathematics, and memorization. Their motto is "Promoting excellence through academic competition." I took the excellence and competition part quite seriously. Picture me hitting the game-winning shot over a taller guard, inking a triple-double that day, while later cornering a couple of wannabe child prodigies with an equation that brought tears to their eyes as I walked away with yet another trophy. In my memory, it's always me crossing the finish line and carrying off the hardware.

I guess in these cases, the finish line didn't actually exist; it was a trophy or mere bragging rights over unsuspecting victims. But my mother didn't care what the hardware was. She just constantly reminded me that I was coming home with the victory.

A passion to compete and win burned deep inside me. It was rooted in showing people I could win, that I could be the best and feel accomplished. Where did this deep longing for academic and athletic supremacy come from? In many ways, I always felt like I was the underdog. I was often a head shorter than all the other basketball players. And I never had the best coaches at the start of academic games tournaments like the kids I competed against.

I needed the trophy for affirmation. Internally, if I didn't win, if I wasn't the best, it ate at me. I would dwell on it until I had another chance to compete and win. If my chance was immediate, we had to have a rematch right then and there. If my chance at a rematch came later, then I couldn't stop thinking about it until I had another shot at getting the trophy, medal, or prize. The internal stakes felt incredibly high, almost as if I was trying to get revenge through competition for what I felt I didn't have. I needed to show whoever was watching that I had what it took. That I was man enough, tall enough, big enough, Black enough, tough enough... simply enough.

As a young kid and up through my marathon days, and even with all the success I achieved academically and professionally, I would compete to prove I was worthy and enough. But with every accolade and every trophy, there was one person who wasn't so convinced that Charles Moore was entirely enough. That person was me.

Would my eventual foray into marathoning and nineteen finishes (more on all that a little later) finally give me the validation I needed? What would happen if I didn't get it? Who would I become? How could I prove to myself and others that I was worthy and more than enough? That I could just be?

^^^

In my first year of middle school, which was also my first year competing in AGLOA, we finished in third place. I was a rookie, but I was clearly the best player on our team and showed promise as one of the top five in the city. We gathered around to discuss our multiple close calls against the two other schools. Each player on our five-person team had won some and lost some nail-biters. "The important thing is that you had fun doing it," our coach said. I wanted no part of that discussion: the emotional participation trophy. I smelled blood and I wanted gold and hardware, not comforting words. Leading into our first state tournament, I remember my mother bringing me to the bus stop. "Go get 'em, son. Just remember, there are individual trophies too," she said. I guess Mom only cared about one person and one person only: me.

This would be the first time I had gone away without my parents. The state tournament comprised the best teams from all regions of Michigan. Teams were bused across the state, arriving in the center of the state to compete for team and individual honors. We didn't know the state tournament would just be a repeat of the regionals. Our team got spanked, and although I won my games, it would not be enough to take the team to the nationals. During those years, I was probably the rare kid in Detroit who was a Michael Jordan fan. As his team was losing in the playoffs on the court, so was mine in the tournament rooms. I returned feeling a bit somber but ready to get back into training mode for next year.

^^^

My parents worked hard and always wanted the best for their children. So, when they had saved up enough money to move to a better neighborhood, they didn't hesitate. I remember coming to school, glowing, knowing I was moving near Sherwood Forest, where all the rich kids lived in the city. I thought my team would be happy for me, but Alicia, one of my teammates, cornered me, asking, "Which bus are you catching to get here?"

Bus? Me? On a bus? Now, why would I do such a thing when I'd be within walking distance of a better school? Which happened to be one of our bitter rivals, the number two school in Detroit. I remember coming home that day unhappy, bitter, and wondering what *team* really meant if my team wasn't happy for me. My mother responded as best she could: she took me shopping.

We prepared as if I had made it to the national tournament. I got a brand-new pair of Air Jordan 5s in white, three pairs of white Jordan shorts, and three white Jordan T-shirts. But for some reason, my mother got a little upset with me when we went to the school clothes section. At this point in my life, I wore nothing but khaki pants, Ralph Lauren and Tommy Hilfiger polo shirts, and Sperrys or Rockports. Mom tried to get me into Levi's jeans. "You don't have to fit in with all your preppy friends!" she barked.

"But Mom, it *is* them. They try to dress like me, not the other way around," I responded. "And besides, if you buy me those Levi's, I won't wear them."

We stormed out of Hudson's department store and drove home in silence. It was our first fight.

My mom had no business calling me preppy. I don't ever remember her driving a car that wasn't a Volvo, and at one point while growing up, she had a sedan and a wagon. She loved her wagon. Her favorite number was 850 because that was the big Volvo sedan. She topped it off with a vanity license plate, FAFNGOD (Faith in God), which she has had since the late eighties. She always straightened her hair, which complemented her high yellow skin, and her most comfortable attire was a monochromatic T-shirt, casual designer jeans, and Sperry's with no socks. She also had a smile that could fill any room, and she found the good in everything.

It was around this time she began going to church. She put

down her packages of cigarettes for Bible verses. Her truth was hers and she didn't need anyone to tell her what to do or how to do it, and if no one wanted to go to church with her, she consistently made her way on her own. I guess that's where I got my ability to be adventurous, along with my tenacity to try new things.

Boarding the charter bus to Atlanta was my first time going out of state without my parents or grandparents. I was twelve. I arrived at the campgrounds in Atlanta, forgetting that I hated insects, pests, and anything dirty. I had come to win every academic game competition put in front of me. Oh, and basketball.

Immediately after dropping my bags off, I noticed the high schoolers playing basketball. I changed into my Jordan 5s and my all-white Jordan outfit and headed over to remind them I wasn't just an equations whiz . . . and a pretty face. As I walked onto the court, someone yelled, "Hey, man, you can't play on the court in all that white gear! It'll get ruined."

The iron oxides and the acidic rain that are prevalent in Georgia create a type of red clay dirt. Contemporary remedies and cleaning advances have made it much easier to clean it out of white clothing. But not in 1989. And of course, not only did my clothes get ruined, but so did my all-white Air Jordan sneakers. *I didn't care.* You couldn't tell me nothing.

At the nationals, I swept the individual awards, bringing home trophies in three different game categories. I tormented the bigger kids, I was faster and smarter on the court, and you couldn't leave me open because my shots were raining. Furthermore, it seemed to be my first foray into fashion because I looked like a Nike ad. I had the most complex equation combinations, a lethal jump shot, and the red stains on my white Jordans didn't stop me from being the best dressed on the court.

That Monday when I returned home, Mom made my favorite dishes for dinner—Chilean sea bass, broccoli, and mashed potatoes. If I drank champagne that young, we certainly would've popped a bottle to celebrate.

"Yeah, that's my son," she said, smiling as my dad and sister looked at us like we didn't even notice them in the room. "I bet none of those kids saw you coming, but they knew who you were once you left. Have faith in God, and He will provide."

When I returned to school that week, I felt a massive void. The euphoria of competition, of winning, of being enough in the moment of victory was gone. Who was I if I wasn't competing and winning? Would it continue to eat away at me? Would I ever be able to outrun this feeling?

Chapter 02

Adrenalin!

I found myself lying in bed, next to my wife, Andrea, staring at the ceiling. The sun blared through the window as forcefully as the drums of the human timekeeper I was listening to, Rock & Roll Hall of Famer Al Jackson Jr. Al died two months shy of age forty. I was age forty.

Last night, I had decided, was the last night I was going to lie lifelessly in bed. My body began to feel peaceful, undisturbed. I'd had my apartment painted the previous week, and the walls of my bedroom were still emanating semitoxic fumes. I felt dizzy, I had a headache, and my eyes watered. But it wasn't my new porcelain-white walls that were doing this to me; it was a nasty cold. The feeling of claustrophobia came over me quickly as the sun's rays beat against my head, not unlike a pair of solid oak drumsticks banging against the head of a snare drum.

Should I lie in bed another day and continue to rest, I wondered, *or relinquish myself from the cycle of restlessness, stillness, and insomnia that has consumed me the last three nights—which already feels like an eternity?*

I'm never sick. But when I am, I simply wait it out. It's the *only* time I rest. Most type A personalities fail at defining and implementing rest in their routine. Freedom from activity? Refraining from labor? My mother once mailed me a handwritten note that read *If your bachelor's degree isn't enough, go get a master's.* But I had already finished my MBA in finance abroad in Rome, Italy. When I glanced out my window now, I imagined that the back of Peter Dillon's 36th pub was the side entrance of Galleria Nazionale d'Arte Antica, where I'd frequently visit to see *Judith Beheading Holofernes* by Michelangelo Merisi da Caravaggio. If only I were still in Rome . . . but I was lying in bed in Midtown Manhattan, and the blaring drums in my head were not Al Jackson beats, but the beatdown that the city of gods gives to the weak.

I'd lived in Italy for several years—from 2009 to 2012, to be exact. I was thinking of those moments, when I was working on my courses in finance in the evenings and taking Italian lessons, visiting museums, and searching the internet for opera or ballet tickets during my days. I didn't know it then, but I wouldn't last very long in finance because there was something intellectually creative brewing inside me.

I changed the music to something a little lighter: a ballet russe mix by Sergei Prokofiev. I played this mix when I wanted to be serene and calm, likely reading a book or studying for some exam. I began to feel like I had just popped a muscle relaxer as I sunk into the bed. My throbbing head was propped up ever so slightly by a pillow, fluffy like the tutus worn by the ballerinas who danced in my head when I managed to get a little sleep. But then the drumming started again, and my heart began to pound. An oboe duet emerged through the speakers and pushed the ballerinas aside, causing my eyes to flicker open for good. I felt the need to rise while André 3000 spit his verse in "Int'l Players Anthem (I Choose You)." I texted my mother to fill her in on my convalescence and then decided that, once and for all, I needed to get out of this house.

The same sun that pierced through my window met me at my front door. I admired the weekend warriors who got to spend their Sunday mornings in Sag Harbor, New York, relishing the morning omelets and Bloody Marys at the American Hotel at 49 Main Street. But instead, I approached Fifth Avenue, returning to my grace, like Jordan making a triumphant comeback with the number 45 on his back. Maybe my comeback wasn't as serious as MJ's, but it felt good to be back in the land of the living and simply walking to get a little air and some food.

As I began my stroll, an odd idea popped into my head: "Charles, we're going to Columbus Circle." I didn't remember ever making this 1.7-mile, thirty-five-minute trek across Central Park. Thankfully, with a little city air on my face, I was beginning to feel better. I popped my headset on and started to scroll through Spotify. The red album cover with a phoenix stuck out—*My Beautiful Dark Twisted Fantasy*—a masterful record by the artist formerly known as Kanye West. *Today is like my own beautiful, dark, twisted fantasy,* I thought after I narrowly missed getting hit by a taxi driver who was texting and driving.

I had always dreamed of living here in New York City. I had eventually made the brash decision in 2005, leaving East Lansing, Michigan, where I had been for the past few years, when I knew it was time to leave. And not just go on vacation, but rather make a change in scenery. Leaving my house this morning was like the adventure I had gone on ten years ago. New York was my town. "It's the magic hour," Ye rapped, addressing this moment. The magic hour, that moment I rounded the corner. *It*, the New York City Marathon that is, has emerged each year on the first Sunday of November for the last forty or so years. Everything slowed as the guitar roared like the speed of light through my headphones, my eyes burst out of my head as I saw hundreds of runners, and even more spectators. The song ended. I cut off the music. I had to listen to the music of HOKAs and Nikes and ASICS pounding the pavement as they rounded the corner to the start of the final eight hundred meters.

I turned to one of the spectators and asked, "What's going on?"

Without actually turning toward me, she replied with an annoyed but pretentious grin, "It's the New York City Marathon." And she returned to form, yelling, "You got this!" to no one in particular.

Apparently, it was marathon Sunday in New York City. My curiosity was sparked. I had walked a 5K in 2006 to support people affected by kidney disease, and just last year, I had gracefully bowed out of a 5K turkey trot in Wilmington, Delaware. I was clueless about what it actually meant to run a marathon; I only knew it was long . . . 26.2 miles long. I tried to visualize the start of the race.

My initial fascination with this race came from looking into the eyes of the would-be finishers. As the yet-to-finish runners bounced around at breakneck speed, those with medals strolled by me gracefully at the speed of a Galápagos tortoise. The stoic calmness of their stroll fascinated me. The experience of seeing runners crossing the finish line at the marathon stimulated my curiosity. I was intrigued by what I saw in the faces of the runners that were distorted by looks of defeat, even in the faces of those crossing the finish line. They had completed the marathon but looked broken and beaten down by the mental and physical feat they had subjected themselves to.

The entire scene moved in slow motion. I had no clue why so much emotion had overtaken me in that moment; God knew I had to walk to this very spot. But I knew then that I was going to run the New York City Marathon—someday. Someday soon.

Chapter 03

My mom always told me I could do anything and be anything.

Ever since I was twelve, I knew that one day, I'd live in New York City and Italy. I used to tell my parents and friends, "I'm going to work on Wall Street someday and learn to speak Italian in Rome." My friends all would laugh and chalk this up as another one of those arrogant, ambitious moments of this weird kid. But my mom always told me I could do anything, be anything, and have everything. And I was crazy enough to listen to her.

I got very close to Wall Street right after high school. I deferred my admission to Michigan State University by a year.

I'd like to say it was because of my internship with Merrill Lynch, but in reality, it was for a girl. I had this girlfriend who was a year younger than me, so I applied for banking jobs as an excuse to stay in town another year. Mom was furious. "You're going to college!" she'd yell at me daily.

I felt she should be happy. It was only months ago I had had her sign papers to get her underage son parental permission to join the US Marine Corps. My father, Derrick, would laugh at her. "You know this boy ain't reporting for military duty. He listens to Tony Bennett, can't get out of bed before ten, and would rather read a book than get his hands dirty," he'd tell her over and over. According to her, she wasn't calling my bluff when those two recruitment soldiers were shoving a stack of papers in her face and she'd cried. "Are you sure you want to do this?" she'd casually ask. "Yes," I'd respond, thinking, *When is she going to tell me I can't?* There was no way I was going into the marines. I had just started dating the girl of my dreams right after graduation.

Eventually, we'd send the marines their walking papers. I'd be making my way to the Merrill Lynch Downtown location, where I'd keep my navy suit—no pun intended. When I was in that office, I felt so much closer to New York City. I read the financial newspapers every day and dreamed about meeting the real-life Gordon Gekko: Carl Icahn or George Soros. My mentor (the only African American in the office) and I would gush over lines from the film *Wall Street*. He'd be Michael Douglas and I, Charlie Sheen, of course. "Money never sleeps, pal," he'd always remind me.

After about a year of working in Downtown Detroit, I'd have to own up to my deferral and eventually enter Michigan State University as a freshman. It seemed like a blur how fast the time went. I remember that one day, I was sitting in my midwestern dorm room, with Frank Sinatra's "New York, New York" blasting from my stereo. I envisioned my future stretching out: days spent making million-dollar deals alongside Gordon Gekko, nights spent with the ladies from *Sex and the City* . . . Hold on a minute. Those people weren't even real. What about the actual people who lived in New York City? What were they like? What was so tough about the city that made it difficult to make it, yet so unique that so many wanted to tough it out?

I eventually got bored with college, dropped out, and worked a series of nonsensical jobs over the next few years. I homed in on my hobbies for intellectual stimulation, which included a range of musical interests, art museums, and literature. Sometime in 2002, I started dating a girl named Flor from Mexico and working as a salesman. We were inseparable. Two or three times a week, she'd bring me lunch and hang out with me on my break.

One such day after lunch, one of my colleagues came up to me and asked, "Wait, she's really from Mexico?"

"Yeah, she's from a town right outside of Mexico City."

"Like, from Mexico . . . so she speaks Mexican?" he asked.

I was stumped. I thought he was joking. "No, buddy, she speaks Spanish. They speak Spanish in Mexico."

He looked about as confused as I was.

Later that night when I got home, I looked at myself in the mirror, thinking, *That guy is about to graduate from college!* I couldn't believe it. *Here I am, a college dropout, and that bonehead is about to graduate.* I jumped online and started looking for the fastest way to a college diploma.

I would start school in 2003. To celebrate, I booked a trip to New York City. I'd always fantasized about living in New

York City. I had three things planned: see Wall Street (easy, since I was staying a block away at Club Quarters Hotel), visit the Metropolitan Opera (I'd recently developed a passion for opera), and go to the 40/40 Club (my favorite rapper at the time was Jay-Z, and he'd recently opened the luxury sports bar).

I called the club to make a reservation and got Desiree Perez on the phone. I had no clue she was one of the club's founders. We talked for almost two hours. I rambled on about how I knew one day I'd be living in the city and what a big Jay-Z fan I was and how I would be there soon. At the end of the call, she said my conversation had moved her. She overnighted me a VIP membership card and told me I'd be on her personal guest list when I arrived. Long before I'd post up after work and have a martini at the King Cole Bar in the St. Regis Hotel, I'd be sitting next to Jason Kidd in the VIP lounge, thanks to a casual yet emotional phone call with a gatekeeper.

^^^

As a child, running is your first lesson in fatigue. As an adult who happens to be a marathon runner, my fatigue comes from knowing that few people who run long-distance footraces look like me.

People have always assumed that I am outgoing and extroverted. Maybe it's my zodiac sign: Leo. I've been told it's my body language: I carry myself with a high level of confidence. Or maybe it's my drive to achieve. The truth is, I am an introvert who occasionally ventures out. In middle school, I was afraid to speak in class, so I broke eye contact whenever teachers would ask questions that I easily knew the answers to. People often say

I have an energy that causes people to gravitate toward me. But social interactions drain that energy from me. I guess because I prefer reading a book or watching a film over being around large groups of people.

On the basketball court, my mouth always got me into trouble, like the time when we moved to a new neighborhood in middle school and within a week, I exerted my will on everyone within a ten-block radius on the basketball court. It was also the first time I almost got beaten up for announcing that I was a superior gamer. My confidence and will to win shadowed my stature and nerdy demeanor. But to be sure, I backed up all the trash I talked with my will to win.

I enjoyed team sports, like basketball and football, but never played on organized teams: only street ball. It makes sense that I would excel in a sport that depends solely upon individual performance, like tennis or golf. I never tried those sports. As a kid, I was too busy toting my attaché case, headed to the weekly AGLOA tournament. I was a naturally curious person. I tried everything from piano, trumpet, hockey, and even dabbled in foreign languages. Imagine my mom's surprise when, in 2005, I began working at 44 Wall Street and, in 2009, I moved to Rome.

My mind always wandered. As an intern at a law office in East Lansing, Michigan, my boss walked into my cubicle and glanced at the book I was thumbing through. "A little light reading there, Charles?" I gave a little smile and went back to perusing Freud's *The Interpretation of Dreams*. Around the same time, I began my self-induced romance with other books by Freud, as well as by Ralph Ellison, F. Scott Fitzgerald, Skip Gates, Jung, Kant, Machiavelli, Marx, Toni Morrison, Nabokov, Nietzsche, Tolstoy, and Cornel West. I'd later develop a slight obsession with famed poet and novelist Charles Bukowski, Chekov, and Brett Easton Ellis, along with a strong dislike for Henry James. Every copy of *The Turn of the Screw*, in my opinion, should be put on haloperidol and then fed to a Euophrys omnisuperstes.

I have always been the person whom people turn to for advice or counsel. My natural instinct is to help others solve problems, to find reflection and space for resolution. My words often encourage people to move forward. Naturally, I'd make a great coach or manager, but I lack the desire to hold that title: "I'm more like Michael Jordan, not Phil Jackson," I'd often lament. Jackson, the head coach of the Chicago Bulls in the 1990s during their six-time championship run, changed Jordan from a premier superstar individual player to a winner. I have an innate desire to be well-rounded and am strongly motivated by winning. As my friend David once said, "You've always wanted that trophy."

My parents had my brother fifteen years after me. I named him because they, oddly, had no clue what to call him. He'd be named II (the second, not Jr.) after his dad, as would my son, almost thirty years later.

When my siblings fight, they call me.

When my friends have relationship issues, they call me.

Sometimes random people who meet me feel that energy, and they ask me questions about navigating the world or life.

I was successful as a financial adviser because a large part of the role was listening to people discuss what was going on in their life and trying to find meaning in it, as well as solving problems with their financial plan.

When I think about those years of informal athletic and formal academic competition, or devouring books by authors from places I had never heard of, it wasn't the trophy I was chasing; it was the adventure, experimentation, and overcoming obstacles. It wasn't the medal (at first) that drove me to run my first marathon, but rather the feeling I saw when I gazed into the runners' eyes. I equated it with how Stevie Wonder must have felt when he carved out the double LP *Songs in the Key of Life*: you have a lot of work to do to get this output. If this all sounds like I'm ranting, then you're right. Another thing I tend to do. Okay, rant over.

^^^

Seeing the runners cross the finish line at the New York City Marathon stimulated my curiosity. So when I was standing at the finish line of the race, I felt like everything else was moving, but in slow motion. You know, like that scene in *The Matrix* on the rooftop. Except I'm not on the veranda. Imagine I'm Keanu Reeves. I'm standing on the corner as if it were the stage of the Bolshoi Theatre, still light-headed, frail, and in need of cobalamin. I imagine ballerinas at their first performance at the Bolshoi, the most prestigious stage for ballet possibly anywhere on the planet. The runners move about like exhausted replicas of Prince Siegfried and Baron von Rothbart (the rivals in *Swan Lake* who compete for the hand of Odette, the Swan Queen). But the runners are not vying for Odette's attention. They're spent, breathless, and not in the mood to break their path. I'm dodging these graceful runners as they glide by me, medals around their necks, faces full of victorious anguish.

But that was yesterday. Today, I'm searching the internet. I don't even really know what a marathon is. Okay, so I know it's a twenty-six-mile race. In a 2009 article for *The Atlantic*, Lane

Wallace pondered questions from marathon elitists. I knew what elitism was. But I had no clue it could be included in the same line as *marathoner*.

Derived from the Latin term *eligere*—a verb meaning "to select" or "to choose"—elitism is rooted in meritocracy. It refers to the exclusivity of a small group of people; the concept is generally used in class systems like the United States, whose democratic society lies in stark ideas that certain groups have greater access to opportunity based on their intelligence, expertise, and experience. While elitism isn't inherently founded in birth or wealth, the notion does reveal that specific demographics are more likely than others to rise to the top or hold positions of power. But what, then, was a marathon, and what were its roots?

It all started (probably) in ancient Greece with Pheidippides, who was a soldier and messenger. When the Persian armies invaded Greece, they met Athenians and Plataeans at the Battle of Marathon. The Greek soldiers were nearing a victory when Pheidippides observed something strange: a single Persian ship had turned away from the fighting. Rather than supporting the soldiers still on the battlefield, the navy was taking an early leave. Pheidippides correctly interpreted this to mean that the Persians intended to use the battle as a distraction and sack Athens while the Greek soldiers were celebrating.

Without a word to anyone, Pheidippides began running. He fled Marathon, running the entire forty-kilometer distance to Athens. Because of his awareness and his endurance, Pheidippides successfully warned the Athenians of the incoming ship and notified them of the Greek victory. He collapsed and died a moment later.

The legend of Pheidippides was enough to inspire the first

marathon race in the original ancient Olympics. This race then became the hallmark event at the 1896 Olympics when Pierre de Coubertin revived them. Since then, events such as the Boston Marathon and the New York City Marathon have given rise to a marathon movement. Today, there are marathons run in every major city worldwide.

So, *I* was going to do that? I was going to run a marathon?

The morning was a bright and sunny day in November 2015. My cold had evaporated, my energy levels were back to normal, and I was just on a nice, casual stroll in Manhattan. Things got a little cloudy for me that afternoon on November 1, because I had no previous interest in running. In 2007, I had walked a 5K to support the National Kidney Foundation and had balked at every turkey trot 5K ever since, including the one I had watched in 2014. I had been fairly athletic as a kid, but I had never run track and had had no inclination to run races at any point in my life. When my father had laughed about me joining the marines, his reaction went something like, "He doesn't like getting up early." Funny enough, most marathons have early-morning starts.

The internet, starting with random Google searches, was of course my first training coach. After processing what I had seen that November near Columbus Circle, I knew I had never had that feeling in my life and I wanted it. I was going to make it happen. No matter how challenging a task, if I set my mind and attention to it, I will complete it. We're talking about the little kid born and raised in the mean streets of Detroit, confidently telling his friends at the age of twelve he would be in Italy learning Italian one day. Which I did.

At this point, I had no clue what elitism in marathoning meant, and at no point in my life had I ever thought race was a barrier to anything I had ever wanted to do. I walked into any room I wanted to, be it the barbecue or the ballet, La Scala or LA Fitness, the American Hotel in Sag Harbor or a Jay-Z concert at Hyde Park.

The question of diversity among runners hadn't crossed my mind yet. When I first considered running, I did not know what I did not know. I did not know what I was getting into physically. I had no stereotypes to consider. The racial component did not dawn on me until my second marathon, which would take place about a year from then. I had not noticed the differences while racing in the New York City Marathon. And how could I? I hadn't even signed up for the United Airlines NYC Half marathon, which would be my first race and only a couple of months away. Can you believe I was going from couch to half-marathon in a few months? The only reason I chose a half-marathon was because I felt three months was all I needed to prepare. I had no clue what that even meant. I just knew I was doing it. My news outlets of choice were Bloomberg, *The Wall Street Journal, The New York Times*, and *The Atlantic*. So Marcus Ryder's piece for *The Guardian* titled "Why don't black people run marathons?" and Jay Jennings's *Runner's World* article "Why Is Running So White?" would not have ever caught my attention.

What did catch my attention in the early months was all the cool gear. I started with sneakers, the familiar brands like Nike, New Balance, adidas, Brooks, and ASICS. But I started to get to know niche brands like Mizuno, and HOKA. I spent countless hours in JackRabbit, talking the ears off the unlucky running geek who got me as a prospective, noncommittal client. I shelled out the $600 for Garmin's wrist gadget, the fēnix 6, because it would make me run faster, of course. I broke in my ASICS GEL-

NIMBUS 18s after passing on their Metaruns. (*Two hundred fifty dollars for running sneakers?* I figured I'd save the extra fifty bucks to put toward some lululemon workout gear.) My new running obsession quickly became an exercise in restraint from shopping.

Chapter 04

Show up.

That morning, of my first half-marathon, cold light beat off the early-winter snow, the powdery ground seeming to beckon the pitter-patter of my ASICS— except I only ran outside on race day. It was a motto I'd largely follow for the next three years. I suggest anyone reading this not to follow my training regimen. I hadn't developed a routine, something that would follow me throughout my running career.

My first order of business as a runner: subject myself to the sticker shock of what Manhattanites deem the bougie gym— Equinox. My street, East Thirty-Fifth, just east of Fifth Avenue, was lined with trees, and the four-block walk was scenic. One of my favorite buildings was 23 Park Ave.

Regal in its time, and today an emblem of what once was, 23 Park Ave. sits at the intersection of East Thirty-Fifth Street and iconic Park Avenue. It is a core part of the Murray Hill neighborhood and an incomparable testament to the genius of the architectural firm McKim, Mead & White. The exterior stands out on the block, drawing attention to the brilliance and artistry of its design. There is much to marvel at when standing beneath its sturdy walls, gazing up at the structure that dates back to the Gilded Age in the 1880s. From any of the wide and arching windows, one can see out onto the decades of history that have passed before this giant. The gaze of Park Avenue is as rich as ever, snugly fit where it stands, much like every other building in Manhattan. Culture and bustle surround it, but in a way remain separate too, the awning of the entryway forming a passage to another place entirely. Here, in the building also known as the Robb House, the luxurious present day makes peace and blends with the sumptuous past. In 1998, New York City recognized 23 Park Ave. as a historic landmark, further solidifying its place in the city's legacy. And I now finally had an excuse to walk by it a few days a week.

Running outside only on race day is nuts. Running on the treadmill is for most people, me included, as entertaining as opening a pile of junk mail after a long vacation. You're running in place in a temperature-controlled setting for thirty minutes or an hour, or maybe even for four hours. Imagine doing that over and over for months leading up to a marathon. I'd quickly run out of Led Zeppelin and Kanye West albums and would resort to watching CNN on one of the many televisions in the middle of the gym. Depressing. Not to mention that the indoors can't emulate the varied terrain and unpredictable weather conditions that one will be certainly subjected to on race day. You will therefore have no experience dodging the spitters, the curbs, or the angry birds just waiting to poop on you. Imagine being inside with the heat at seventy-four degrees and then walking outdoors, missing your Canada Goose jacket in freezing temperatures. Yeah, it's about as traumatizing as the $185 bill for my first month at the bougie gym.

When I started training for my first half-marathon, I ignored all the rules. I happen to have a morbid dislike for rules, disorganized kitchens, hairy people, holidays (I forget the dates anyway), the color purple (not the film), and restaurants that start with the letter A. They only do that to be listed first in the yellow pages. In fact, when it comes to gathering with large groups of people, I'm the winner of the Charles Bukowski award. Bukowski would say, "Wherever the crowd goes, run in the other direction. They're always wrong." So why am I running a marathon that attracts so many disorganized, hairy rule followers . . . and just lots of people in general?

I am originally from Detroit—the Motor City. We Detroiters know cars and never have a hard time getting our hands dirty. Well, most of us. I prefer to work with my head rather than my hands. My grandfather, always the hard worker, toiled in the coal mines of North Carolina before moving to Detroit for employment in the automobile industry. He tried to instill in me the importance of working hard and the only way he knew how—working with your hands.

When I was in middle school, he called me to the front of his car one day. He wanted to teach me about the care and maintenance of an automobile. I said, "I'm not going to need this. I'll pay someone to do it."

My grandfather looked at me strangely. I thought he was going to sling a torque wrench at me. Luckily, he was against violence. All that to say, it is totally out of character for me to aspire to run for four or five hours with a gaggle of maniacs.

I worked out for three months preparing for the 2016 United Airlines NYC Half marathon. I had no clue what I was doing or how to prepare. I just knew running was required. In the beginning, I went to the Equinox gym, already in gear since I hated gym locker rooms, and headed straight to the treadmill. In hindsight, I should have googled a training plan online, but I was a little stubborn and just really thought it was going to be a cakewalk.

The first day, I ran one mile. Over the next few weeks, I'd pop into the gym for about an hour; I'd stretch and run for one to three miles per visit. After a few weeks of that, I increased the daily mileage to around three to four miles per visit. Ultimately, I capped out at six miles—once.

During training, I was always dehydrated. I couldn't drink the water fast enough, or maybe the amount I was drinking was insufficient. My body constantly felt like an iris; I not only tolerated copious amounts of water, I needed it. A far cry from what the recommended training may be. This would require you to build up to around ten miles before tapering off, decreasing the mileage run shortly before the race, and then running the half-marathon. I seriously thought I was doing something productive. I came home after every visit, showered, dressed, got ready for work, and started telling everyone I knew I was training for a half-marathon.

I had to tell everyone I knew because the only way for me to get into this race was to raise money for charity to guarantee my entry. So I went to the only place I knew I could throw the idea out there and not face rejection in person: Facebook. Then I selected a charity I'd support: the National Multiple Sclerosis Society. There are a few reasons why I chose this charity. First,

I had volunteered on their Young Professionals Committee for a couple of years when I had first moved to New York City, and Michelle—a close friend of my wife, Andrea—battles the disease every day. There were other charities, but I felt the most connected to this one.

The deal for the charity run goes as follows: You register for the popular race as early as possible—spots do get filled—and guarantee yourself a bib/race number; in return, you commit to raise a set amount of money, which is tax deductible for the people who support you, and the funds go to that charity. In this case, I had to raise $1,500 for multiple sclerosis, and I'd be in. Raising the money was surprisingly easy. I think most of my sponsors felt sorry for me. My friends all knew I'd rather be browsing the aisles of the Strand bookstore so I could peruse a Colson Whitehead novel rather than dashing down Fifth Avenue or through Central Park looking like a wannabe superhero in tights. Who would put themselves through running 13.1 miles for fun? I guess me.

I had no clue it was to be this cold in mid-March. Never being accustomed to the cold even though I'm from Michigan, I looked at the weather app on my iPhone, and a huge 33 appeared. But I was excited to run my first race. I woke up early, dusted off my sneakers, and put on the outfit I had laid out the night before: black ASICS, matching black running tights, a dusky T-shirt with matching gloves and hat, and an onyx jacket. I looked like I was ready to prance around Newport, Rhode Island, in off-peak season, still drowsy from the previous evening's oysters and old-fashioned cocktails at Clarke Cooke House.

Starting out in Central Park, the 2016 United Airlines NYC Half marathon looped upward before descending through

Midtown Manhattan, then toward the Hudson River side of the city and down along the west side of Manhattan, ending in an emotional spiral to the finish line on Wall Street. I was about to finish my first race: a half-marathon. It was magnificent for encompassing some of the best sights that New York City has to offer for a marathoner.

I crossed the finish line with a joy I didn't know was possible. And I had also found a way to practice running for a marathon without subjecting myself to the monotony of the treadmill: running shorter races outdoors. Back home, I whipped open my MacBook and began searching for more races on the New York Road Runners (NYRR) website. I signed up for and ran the UAE Healthy Kidney 10K, which was extremely emotional and sentimental. My dad had gained his angel wings in the fall of 2010 while I was off galivanting around the world, living in Rome, Italy. Plaguing African Americans at high rates, chronic kidney disease was what took my dad.

According to some of the most recent statistics, African Americans make up approximately 13 percent of the United States population but constitute approximately 35 percent of those experiencing kidney failure in this country. The rates of diabetes and high blood pressure remain high in the African American community, and kidney failure naturally follows. Even when chronic kidney disease is treatable, it still introduces a range of ills and complications.

Some of the most common symptoms of chronic kidney disease are weight loss, shortness of breath, and tiredness, all of which substantially affect overall quality of life. African Americans experience kidney failure at a rate nearly three times of the general population, and we need to research and better understand the impact it is making on African American families every day.

While kidney disease and its root causes are treatable, it can rapidly become untreatable. The cost of such a progression is the highest that any family can pay. Every year, approximately 52,000 people die from nephritis or a related ailment, which involves the slow and painful deterioration of the flesh, a fate from which we need to protect more people through awareness and research initiatives for dialysis access and ongoing kidney research. Other initiatives may look at genetic testing to determine risk factors earlier and more accurately, and to promote preventive measures for lowering blood pressure.

My dad was a hard worker and a culinary god. But most of all, he loved his family and would protect them with his own life. His love for basketball, both playing and spectating, permeated his early years. As undeviating as his work ethic on the courts at Oakland Community College where we often balled and rising through the ranks at culinary steakhouses and Italian eateries, he was just as fierce in front of a plate filled with the carnal delights. His taco salads with salad bowls from scratch were my favorites. But what I miss most from him is his ability always to offer words of encouragement and never discount any of the crazy dreams of grandeur I had. He was always my biggest fan ... after my mother, of course. In his final years, before he got really sick, we became close friends. We discussed everything. My fondest memory was him expressing his admiration for my big dreams and my commitment to them. It meant a lot hearing such encouragement directly from him.

Anyway, Bib #4745—yours truly—darted through Central Park and, with a pace of 10:47 minutes per mile, I crossed the finish line and sent a blessing up high for him. My outdoor training was truly enjoyable as long as there was a starting and a finish line.

^^^

I didn't like running. Mornings were a drag and getting up early to go to spend it on a treadmill instead of in a coffee shop with an Ethiopian "pour over" and a Marlon James novel hadn't yet become my idea of a good time. I hated sweating, so I avoided most activities that raised my body temperature too high. I remember one morning shortly after running the United Airlines NYC Half marathon, trying my hardest to get back to training, I started making up excuses in my head. *What if I get hit by a car walking to the gym? Don't I have extra work to do? I don't have time for the gym. I think I hear Mom calling.* None of this changed the fact that if I wanted to run the New York City Marathon in November, I had to keep on training and running; waking up early was just a by-product of what needed to be done. "At least you look cute in all your lululemon gear," Andrea said. "Yeah, okay, there is that," I agreed.

Andrea was one of my true inspirations who had led me to get into running (the other being my uncle Jr.) and had been running most of her adult life. We met in 2008, just before I was leaving for Italy. We kept in touch and remained close until my return to New York City in 2012. We began officially dating shortly afterward and were married in the fall of 2013.

Andrea ran for fun and to maintain good physical fitness. She had run a few races, 5Ks and 10Ks, and had competed in the 2010 New York City Marathon. I'd had no clue, as I had been too busy stuffing my face with pasta and pizza in Italy's capital. Unfortunately, she was pulled off at the sixteen-mile mark due to an abundance of caution. The carb-filled meal from dinner the night before was littered all over the intersection of First Avenue and East Sixtieth Street. She had once told me she had been devastated in that moment, and I could only imagine how angry I'd feel if I was in that position. She hadn't been running for the glory, though; it had been for the love of the running community.

I received advice from everyone—from novice to highly experienced, and even an ambitious never-before-marathoner— it didn't make any difference. I started showing up at every race on the NYRR calendar, but even that wasn't enough. Enter the Tough Mudder, which was a drastic step for me. I've never been a fan of getting dirty, being dirty, or even the word *dirty*. (I still haven't seen the music video to Christina Aguilera's 2002 hit "Dirrty"; I'm nothing if not incredibly consistent.)

The Tough Mudder, one of the most beloved obstacle course-style races in the world, is an event unique in its message: come here to test yourself to see how much strength is in you, to understand how far out into the distance you need to venture to find your true limitations. Whether it features thirteen obstacles or thirty, every Tough Mudder is a one-of-a-kind adventure.

I was certain to get dirty. How would I handle it? There would be physical and mental obstacles for me to overcome. Initially, I thought these races, including the marathon, were merely physical challenges. But I would soon find out just how mentally challenging running is as well. Could I rise to the occasion?

This first obstacle race was about getting into the mud and proving I could endure it. Exposure therapy involves exposing people, in a safe context, to a space or situation that is the source of their fear, anxiety, or limiting thought. Identification of a core need, often unrelated to the aversion or compulsion, is critical to the process. The first stage of addressing the challenge is to be present—to show up. The only way to address it—whatever *it* is—is to meet it head-on. I realized I was living in fear of getting dirty. Remember Bill Murray as Bob Wiley in *What About Bob?* or Jack Nicholson as Melvin Udall in *As Good As It Gets*? Well, not quite that bad, but I was just short of needing to consult my local Upper West Side analyst. Of course, it was just all in my head; I lived in New York City. I only realized that limiting thought as I found a way to address it head-on for the achievement of greater life goals. My first step was to suit up and show up.

I can't lie. I thought about self-sabotage. Who would know or care if I didn't show up? What if I injured myself on the way or my transportation canceled on me? The race was on Long Island, and the Long Island Railroad (LIRR) often breaks down—at least, that's what I told myself. I had only ridden the LIRR a total of six times in my entire life, which pretty much qualifies me as an expert on the matter. Maybe. Is it me, or does it smell like hyperbole in here?

Before that first Mudder, I was sure there were runners who meant well and went out drinking the night before, only to awaken hungover from the unfathomable amounts of hefeweizen and Monkey 47 martinis (it was that last one that did it) that would make them skip the race. My self-sabotaging moment never actually occurred, but I may have fantasized once or twice about what would happen if I came down with a bout of temporary paralysis, anything to have an excuse to excuse myself. Or if I popped a few bottles of champagne with friends—the perfect persuasion I needed to opt out.

I still wasn't exactly convinced about the Mudder, though. What was the point? When during the New York City Marathon would I have to swim through sludge to climb a rope out of a ditch or leap over a bale of hay? (*Maybe* at the south end of Central Park near the stable where they kept the carriage horses?) I guess what I'm actually asking is: How would this simulate the environment that I would be in on race day? Uneven terrain, traffic, potholes, and grass were nonexistent on the treadmill. But so was using my hands as windshield wipers to remove wet soil from my face.

It turned out that the Tough Mudder was relatively easy for me. They're actually meant to be fun if you don't mind getting dirty. There are even a lot of corporate teams and group runs. Its rise in popularity occurred simultaneously with the increased popularity of CrossFit workouts. Nevertheless, here I was, pumping my fist as I popped out of the mud like Apollo Creed meets Swamp Thing.

These shorter races early in my running career showed how easily I could become addicted to immediate rewards, much like my college career. With every course and examination, I grew one step closer to obtaining my degree. The immediate rewards in endurance sports come from the activation of your best self to endure the training and implement the discipline. All the smaller races were like courses and exams that moved me closer to my senior thesis, which was the full marathon. Graduation would only come after the finish line. Training does not excite me. But I am excited about crossing the starting line, enduring the punishment of a race, breaking the plane at the finish, and being rewarded with a carved trinket made of synthetic metal alloy attached to a string.

My reign on top as a Tough Mudder was shorter than a leprechaun. I lasted one race. I just didn't see the point. It was too much fun, and it didn't feel like I was preparing myself enough for the challenges of a marathon. Then I heard about Spartan Races. They're like Tough Mudders for iron men. It is about strength, agility, and versatility. The obstacles are extremely challenging. For example, one involves carrying a fifty-pound boulder one hundred feet, dropping for five burpees, and then carrying the boulder back again. I watched a few YouTube clips, and I was instantly hooked. I decided I was going to finish a Spartan Race trifecta before embarking on the New York City Marathon.

Chapter 05

Commit to your unbreakable journey.

Nothing epitomizes getting beaten down, the wind knocked out of you, and still winning than Game 5 of the 1997 NBA Finals. I'm talking, of course, about the flu game. Six years later, the man who had willed himself to dominate during the flu game, a tall, decorated athlete named Michael Jordan, retired for the final time at age forty. Here I was, ready to run my first full marathon at the same age. It was now the summer of 2016. I'd turn forty in August and run the New York City Marathon in November. Just the thought of it should've brought fear into my heart—but I didn't know what I didn't know yet.

I needed to push myself like MJ did in that iconic game. If the Tough Mudder was a fun ride, the Spartan Race would be an exercise in the futility of chaos. When I first looked out at the course, it seemed almost fanciful. *I just did the Tough Mudder obstacle course. This can't be too much more daunting . . . can it?* Taking in those mind- and back-breaking obstacles, I couldn't help but picture someone wandering out onto them after race day and climbing atop them the way a cat would a new tower toy. Yet they are not toys, nor is the course fanciful in any traditional sense of the word. That much becomes clear very quickly the first time you take on a Spartan Race.

The Spartan Race is just different: one must experience it to fully grasp it. The first leg is the Spartan Sprint. The length of this leg will vary, but at a minimum, you can expect to run three miles. On average, most Spartan Races will require you to run five miles if the course is outdoors. Here is the caveat: It is not five miles of flat ground. It is not five miles of hills either. Instead, you will cover between three and five miles of obstacles. There are an average of twenty or so obstacles across the Spartan Sprint, which means that you should be able to breeze through a regular 5K or 10K before you take on this first leg of the trifecta. *I wish I knew this beforehand,* I thought. But honestly, I have no clue if I would've listened or done anything differently. So here I was, driving out to Pennsylvania to run with the Spartans.

The first canto of these races was like an intro or prelude, and the morning of July 16, 2016, was a scorcher. It was ninety-five degrees in the mountains of Palmerton, Pennsylvania, and standing at the top of Blue Mountain, I felt as if I were only a few inches from the sun. The heat is not my friend. I stay inside when it is extremely hot. My body does not respond well; exhaustion is inevitable when I am in the sun too long. There were a couple of thousand people there crazy enough, or as unbriefed as I, taking on this feat.

Enduring that experience over the course of two hours was an immense challenge. A twenty-yard bear crawl beneath barbed wire up the mountain was one obstacle. Your back could be shredded if you rose too high. The mountain's steep and pebbly ground also serves as a heater of sorts in the oven of the environment.

After reaching the top of the mountain, about halfway through the race, I encountered a gentleman in his late twenties, probably around six feet one and about 175 pounds. I took this as a great opportunity to rest; I was exhausted, and my heart rate was as high as that mountain and searing like the tuna in a niçoise salad. My "It'll all work out on race day" training was starting to show: amateur hour. He, on the other hand, looked a lot like former star NFL wide receiver Terrell Owens. I never relish the pain of others, but I had a slight feeling of relief when I noticed that even he was having a hard day. As we pressed forward side by side for a few minutes, we discussed the different levels of the Spartan Races.

"Why did you do this one—the hardest one—as your first?" he asked with a mischievous grin.

"The timing worked out. I'm going for the trifecta," I said, beaming with a confidence that belied my incredibly fatigued physical state. "I signed up for the Boston Super and the Killington Beast."

He glanced over at me, looked down in deep thought for a moment, then responded, "The Killington Beast? Take a lot of supplies. I competed last year and failed. I'll be there too."

To hear that this man—a near-perfect physical specimen in his mid- to late twenties—had not completed the race made me question myself. I had no idea what I was in for. It was the first time I had a race on my calendar and doubts about finishing.

The Boston Super, which also took place in mid-August, didn't come with any divine love sent by the Virgin Mary. The second canto of the Spartan Race was even hotter than Palmerton. My email inbox was flooded with warnings from the race administrators:

Race day is almost here. It is predicted to be extremely hot this weekend of our Boston Super Weekend event. For everyone's safety... START HYDRATING. NOW. We STRONGLY recommend that all racers carry a hydration source of at least 32 oz AND an electrolyte source. Wear waterproof sunscreen. If you have concerns about competing in the event, you should consult your physician. But bring it on! Aroo!

And side effects include dizziness, confusion, nausea, vomiting, and an altered mental state. What was this, the black-box warning label for Lexapro?

The Boston Super is, as you can imagine, a step up from the first leg, pushing you that much more. At a minimum, you can expect to run 7.7 miles on a Spartan Super, though lengths up to eleven miles are common. The Spartan Super usually spans just under nine miles. But remember, you are not simply running that length. Because this is the Spartan Race, you are going to face many obstacles. Fortunately, the increase in obstacles is not equivalent to the increase in the length of the race. On average, a Spartan Super features 24.5 obstacles.

When I arrived at the race that morning, my head was spinning. I had just run this crazy obstacle course on a mountain in excruciating heat. One of the side effects from that was, I'll admit, a little bit of fear. These racers looked like they had been doing CrossFit, suitably preparing them for the lifting, tossing, carrying, and climbing. I had only prepared for the running.

If this were a chess match, Mr. Spartan would be yelling, "Checkmate!" by the time I reached the second obstacle.

The heat got to me right away. Sometimes, when I'm out in the sun too long, I get so exhausted that I have to go home and take a nap. I figured if that happened here, I'd have to tap out of the race. I had a racing hat to cover my head, and I wore waterproof sunscreen. Even so, I began dealing with the pressures of the heat right away. I hadn't packed any hydration source, but when I got to the aid stations, I drank like a Gobi Desert camel discovering a new water source. It was tough. It was grueling. The way I beat my chest after I crossed the finish line, you would've thought I had just finished a marathon. I had finished a Spartan Race Super.

I survived. And a few months later, I arrived in Killington, Vermont, to take on the Beast. When I arrived at Ben & Jerry's home state the first night, I was a mess. There was no ice cream. The air was crisp. The evening was long. Imagining I'd get food poisoning from even crackers and water that Saturday evening night before the race, I decided to eat nothing. So literally, the night before running *the* Beast, I decided to eat nothing? Trained musicians probably have a sleep regimen that curbs anxiety the night before a performance. Well-rehearsed politicians and keynote speakers likely sleep like babies before the big speech. Meanwhile, I was having nightmares of Terrell Owens hovering over me like a beast at the starting line, yelling, *"Lasciate ogni speranza, voi ch'entrate!"* (Abandon all hope, ye who enter!) My stomach was growling from the emptiness it felt and every noise I heard had to be a wolf at my door, so the slightest sound reminded me of all my insecurities I had about what would be. I soon woke from that anxious state and faced another—it was time to overcome a beast of a different kind. (And yes, I sometimes daydream in Italian.)

The Beast, which rounded out the trifecta, had a notorious obstacle in the middle of the race ominously called the Death March, which scared even the toughest athlete. This race starts at 6:30 a.m., releasing waves every fifteen minutes of two hundred and fifty runners. It includes a strict midrace cutoff, where if you do not reach the eleventh mile by a certain time, you're deemed a safety risk to yourself and pulled off the course. These races are not for most people. The Beast had a fairly high did-not-finish (DNF) rate, even though everyone there looked as if they'd been training for it all their lives. The women had biceps like famed CrossFit athlete Samantha Briggs and the agility of award-winning triathlete Gwen Jorgensen. The men had the toughness of six-foot-five NFL defensive end J.J. Watt and the brute force of massive New Zealand rugby player Kieran Read.

And then there was me. I consistently undertrained and was more dedicated to reading French literary giant Marcel Proust than to the training techniques of author and marathoner Hal Higdon. As hard as the athletes train, the Spartan Beast is such an immense challenge that it may be too much for even superhuman athletes. This leg of the trifecta averages 13.5 miles and often spans sixteen. The obstacles increase to an average of 28.5, with a minimum of twenty-five. But nothing is more terrifying than the Death March: cue the part in the scary film that begins with nightmarish music.

In Vermont every year, the boldest and the most conditioned meet for the Death March. This obstacle is sure to make even UFC mixed-martial arts fighter Holly Holm rethink her training. Here, competitors will march a mile straight upward on a dirt trail, the elevation change increasing by a foot or more with every step. While a mile may not seem like much, the elevation wears down your legs and lungs: it will browbeat even the most seasoned athletes. I counted thirteen grown men and women shedding tears along the way. The weather, alternating between unforgiving heat and punishing wind, made the march all the more difficult.

The obstacles are, of course, what make the Killington Beast Death March what it is. They number thirty to thirty-five. (They never tell you in advance.) They range from bear crawling underneath barbed wire up a hill, to carrying a giant-size boulder X number of yards, to scaling a one-hundred-foot wall. And then there's the Death March. I have heard among those who have finished it that nothing can prepare one for the pain and doubt that creep in toward the end of that first mile. Yet after that, there is still an entire obstacle course to take on, more pressing and more complex than all others.

The eleventh-mile marker cutoff appeared right before we were rewarded with this crazy obstacle. Alongside the Death March, to the right, one might notice the ski lift going up and down and the spectators lounging in their chairs, gazing at us as we're *punished* for *making* the cutoff. The faces on my fellow racers were of exhaustion. No one ran. We all marched, taking frequent breaks to curve off the pressure. Around halfway up, I started focusing on the spectators, trying to direct my mind elsewhere from the pain of climbing. Andrea had been trailing me along the race, following my every move on the Spartan Race app. Suddenly, I heard my name being called. Andrea yelled, "Charles, I've been looking for you!"

Almost in unison, a few climbers yelled back, "He's a little busy right now!"

As if the climb wasn't bad enough, coming down was brutal on your knees. At every step, you're using a different set a muscles to brace yourself to keep from tumbling down the hill. *If only there was a golf cart to bring me down,* I thought. The bottom of the hill has a base camp like when climbing Mount Everest.

The weather wasn't the problem for me. The terrain was much less forgiving. I'd been running for over six hours before it started to get dark. It was now around 5 p.m., and I was literally running in the woods, in the dark, with a little flashlight on my head, through what felt like the most inhospitable place on Earth with no aid station in sight. For this, you've either packed well, or you may succumb to hunger and resort to munching on poisonous flora. The heavy footsteps and cries around you belong not to ravenous animals but to unlucky athletes who slipped on rock debris or tapped out despite knowing they were so close to the finish.

I was about seven hours in when I hit the wall. I was physically drained. My legs didn't work anymore. Every step felt like, well, I had just ran a marathon. I thought about giving up for a moment. I wondered where the closest medical tent or aid station was, or just someone with a four-wheeler to drive me back to my hotel. I had given it my all and had nothing left in the tank. I stopped. It was pitch black at this point, and my headlamp bled through the forest like a hand parting mist. I knew why my fellow Spartans with the chiseled bodies of Roman soldiers were crying. I had beat the Sprint. I had conquered the Super. I had rented a car and driven all five hundred miles to and from. The Airbnb had been rented. I had paid the $150 registration fee. There was no museum or theater or friend or monument to see in Killington, Vermont. No Michelin-star restaurant to experience. All in, this was a $1,500 trip. If you include the Sprint and Super, I was out around $2,500. I was not leaving this mountain without getting my money's worth. Carrying the head of this beast in my hands like a true Spartan would be a return on my investment.

^^^

To finish it is to know the mind of the warrior, which is the point of the Spartan Race. As the organizers say, "Commit to your unbreakable journey." Venture past the juncture where sense and reason give way to heart and soul, feel the burn, and believe that the finish line is somewhere up ahead.

Grit your teeth. Tuck in your shirt. Grin and bear it. There are so many ways to say that someone is tough, but much more importantly, when you say someone is tough, there may be multiple definitions of the word. Perhaps you are saying that someone can withstand a giant force. They are tough because their muscles are developed, and their heart and lungs can keep on ticking when others have long given up. On the other hand, you may be saying that someone is tough in that they never give up, even after all their organs have cried out and every other instinct but one is telling them to stop.

To cultivate both: That is the secret. Push the body and the mind. Goad each one on in its own way. For the body, look at the length of the trail ahead. Know that unless you prepare for it and unless your body can finish that trail without too much effort, you are not going to get the most out of yourself. Forget about all doubts in your mind and give up on the little games from here on out, simply knowing that, true or not, you are going to believe in your own invincibility. You must. There is no other choice.

Only then is toughness yours—whatever anyone may mean and however they want to describe it in you. Physical and mental toughness can coexist, and when they do, they complement each other, each one becoming that much more impactful. I am a Spartan Trifecta finisher. *Aroo!*

Chapter 06

My Kind of Tribe.

Almost exactly a year before I was born, Diana Ross recorded the theme song to the film *Mahogany*, "Do You Know Where You're Going To?" Do you know where you're going? To outsiders, only your movement is apparent, but the direction never is. You know, though. You know whether you are running toward something or maybe away from it. That knowledge, that inner sense, is the only thing that matters. It is no one else's business whether you are fleeing or pursuing, exiting or entering, on a path going north or south, east or west. You owe no one an explanation.

I'll ask again: Do you know where you're going? You should. Every time you run, ask yourself that question. Reflect on your truth about this direction or that one to understand yourself— and to make sure you are aware of what the finish line looks like and how you want to feel when you get there. Less than a minute into the song, Ross demands of the listener, "What are you hoping for?" When I graduated from Cass Technical High School in 1994 (also the alma mater of Ross), I had no clue what I was hoping for or where I was going. There must be something that draws me to new beginnings and adventures because that sentiment paralleled my feelings leading up to the first of my nineteen marathons.

When I approached the New York City Marathon Expo one November day in 2016, I was overwhelmed. Imagine walking into the Jacob Javits Center, all eight hundred and fourteen thousand square feet of it, and seeing thousands of people lunging for the latest gear—shoes, shirts, shorts, socks. Oh, and to retrieve their race packet. The race packet includes your bib, safety pins, and all the information you need to know to get to the starting line. The expo is also full of all sorts of other information. There are experts who will renounce those without proper running form, style, etiquette, or plan. There is the guy who will sell you a plaque with your medal, picture, and name on it (shipped to you later, of course). There are myriad options of chews and supplements that one may want to pack for the race. Then there are all the vendors carrying the heavy equipment, like massage guns and post-race compression recovery boots. If you're not overwhelmed already, you'll surely lose your mind looking at all the apparel and trying to find your way out.

If the asperity of the expo isn't enough, now you must run the 26.2 miles that comprise the full course. The New York City Marathon is the largest in the world in terms of the number of runners: around fifty thousand. About 30 percent to 40 percent are female, and 60 percent to 70 percent are men. The national average for African American marathon finishers is around 1 percent, and given the fact this race is very international, I imagine those numbers aren't too far off.

I felt I was ready, but I didn't really know exactly what I was getting into that morning. I'd later realize that the weather was near perfect, forty-five to fifty-five degrees, but I was just glad it wasn't ninety. I wasn't nervous, mostly because I didn't know what to be nervous about.

I approached the starting line like a young Mike Tyson doing his prefight stare down of an opponent. I was ready to take a bite out of this marathon. I had already run four half-marathons—5Ks, 10Ks, and Tough Mudders—and was a Spartan Race Trifecta finisher. I had overcome the Killington Beast, conquering the Death March. I had gotten muddy, bloody, and pushed myself beyond what I had thought I was physically capable of. After all that, what obstacle would be insurmountable in this race?

My race started around noon. Out of Wave 4, Corral E came Bib #65610. I wore a custom-stitched black lululemon shirt with my first name emblazoned on the front in white letters. My running tights were black with a gray X on the side by CW-X. The CW-X brand boasts an exoskeletal support of the joints that also helps improve the body's natural movement when running. Lululemon is just comfortable. And, of course, I had already broken in my ASICS GEL-NIMBUS 18s.

Out the gate, I was hot. I was ready to thrust my body past the starting line and finish in a flash. When I stepped into the crowd of overachieving amateur athletes, a realization kicked in that the most I had prepared for this race was my music playlist. I hadn't run the recommended twenty-mile-long run during my training. The farthest I'd run was during the Beast, which was just over a half-marathon. The only guarantee was Kanye West would kick off my first miles. Earlier that year, writer Dorian

Lynskey described him as "a brilliant madman who speaks and acts in superlatives." West's album *The Life of Pablo* had recently dropped, and the critics jumped at his honesty about debts and insecurities in Saint Pablo. I saw it as the foreshadowing of his ascent to billionaire status. Jay-Z's *Magna Carta... Holy Grail* had been out for three years, but for me, it was the most recent version of Jay-Z's evolution as an individual that realized his greatest fantasies. As he raps over the hard-hitting beat—"Jeff Koon balloons, I just wanna blow up"—I imagine his living room resembling the Tate Modern. Hip-hop legend Tupac Shakur had been dead twenty years by the time I made my playlist for this race in 2016. I included a couple of songs from Pac's final album, *Makaveli*, made before his life was tragically taken from him. "Hold Ya Head" is raw. I ended the list with 50 Cent, merely because it felt right to include an artist with NYC roots.

The marathon gods warn you about mile one: *"Don't come out with blazing speed when you're crossing that Verrazzano-Narrows Bridge,"* I'd heard over and over. I'm built for endurance, not sprinting. It typically takes me a couple of miles to warm up. As I entered Brooklyn and made my way past Bay Ridge, I felt like this was going to be a smooth race. In fact, I was cruising down Fourth Avenue, crushing mile after mile along the way. The crowd went wild. No one prepares you for the abundance of cheers one receives during the New York City Marathon. I could only imagine that what I was experiencing was akin to what Kobe Bryant felt while playing and winning in Los Angeles for all those years. Every cheer along the race route felt like it was meant exclusively for me. At this point, my name was covered by my jacket, so in my head, the hoorays were sent just to me.

When I think of that day, I don't think of the dark moment that juxtaposed my initial excitement when I caught the first sight of familiar faces at mile eight. I had been texting with Andrea all morning, and by now, it was early afternoon. As I was passing Flatbush Avenue, I noticed her and her mother, Arline, just before the mile marker. As I approached, I held up one finger and magniloquently dropped for ten pushups. I don't think I had read or heard anyone say that was a good idea, but I guess I was continuing to break the unwritten rules in more ways than one. Not my finest moment of the race. Luckily, I sprung up without ruining my first full marathon with an early injury and dashed to give them hugs.

Andrea asked, "How is the race going? You look great."

Before I could answer, Arline chimed in with, "You look like you're flying through!"

Of course, even if I hadn't been doing well, I would've said I felt great. But in that moment, I felt fantastic. Why else would I be so boisterous so early in the race? Nonetheless, I relieved myself of my jacket and gave it to Andrea to hold—it was starting to get warm—and I was off to the races again. Plus I had to show off my name embroidered on the front of my shirt.

Less than one-quarter of a mile later, I was met by my brother Derrick, or DJ, as he has been called all his life to distinguish him from our father. He had been trying to reach Andrea and Arline before me so we could all gather together, but he had missed the initial reunion by minutes. Of course, I stopped and high-fived him. We chatted for a minute as he lamented about the traffic from one side of Brooklyn, where he lived, to here in Fort Greene.

I soon rounded mile marker sixteen and made a mental note: *This is where Andrea found her limit,* I thought. This small success was a victory for the household. If I knew her, she would have probably said that this incremental victory was the finish line, not mile seventeen. Yet for me, every race had a race within the race. I always counted even the smallest victories—they helped my mental state in completing the larger goal. Finishing is not a grand gesture of completion. Finishing is the culmination of all the small victories.

If the New York City Marathon is where the world comes to run (participants travel from over 140 countries), then First Avenue is where you see how much of a melting pot Manhattan is. At around Sixtieth Street, the spectators became six to ten rows deep. An electrical surge of energy vibrated my entire body. Upon arrival, my heart was racing so much that I had to slow to a walk to allow the vibrancy to enter my soul. I watched as hundreds of runners passed me, and yet the crowd cheered only for me. "Charles, go! You got this, Charles!" It made me feel like I was an athlete known all over the five boroughs. My name just happened to be tattooed on my shirt. The signs hovered over the crowds as people attempted to get the attention of their ponies in the race.

Around mile seventeen, I noticed a familiar face—Anthony, a fellow St. John's grad, who was also walking, but for different reasons. We began talking, and I quickly realized he wasn't doing so hot. "What are you doing here, Charles?" he asked in stoic surprise. He looked beaten down. Exhausted. Battered and bruised from the sixteen miles he had battled through.

"I'm taking a bite out of a twenty-six-mile race," I swung back confidently.

"If I can just reach my family on mile eighteen, I'll get energized," Anthony muttered through labored breaths.

At the time, it didn't cross my mind how important it was that I accompanied him for the next mile till we came upon his tribe; I just did it. It didn't cross my mind until a few marathons later how important community is to the success of something that seems so *individual* focused. We chatted about our training and the race. Mostly I felt the comfort of not just a familiar face but of someone facing an uphill battle alongside me, facing the prospect of failure just as I was. I listened over the screams and cheers; the ground shaking from the spectators' roars echoed the tremble in Anthony's voice. I felt the burst of energy as it leaped inside his body when his family embraced him; he was supercharged. He was at least ten years younger than I and looked as fit as a fiddle. But only a half mile into our reboot, his soul began to flounder again. He needed to walk. As I walked by his side, I was beginning to feel a cramping in my calves that started to seep into my thighs. I knew at that moment it was time to get back into my race. The crisp air didn't help much; I needed to warm my body up again, and there was only one way to do that—start running.

As I entered the Bronx, a brief silent area encouraged me to restart my music. "I don't know what you heard about me," 50 Cent rapped in "P.I.M.P." Even after the song ended, that line danced in my head. Who did the marathon gods think I was? What had they heard about me? If those gods thought for one moment that I wasn't here to get my medal . . . they had been sadly misinformed.

People come out from all over as a community to support the runners. The marathon goes through all five boroughs with thousands of participants and draws more than one million spectators. But there is a point in this northernmost New York City borough where you must remind yourself that the twenty-mile marker is the emotional halfway point, and hopefully you left gas in the tank to finish. My muscles were just starting to warm up, like a forty-year-old car that hadn't been started in years but still had a little juice left. I kept telling myself there was only a 10K left. But at my pace, that meant another hour.

For most of the race, I had also been texting with my mom and Uncle Jr. They're both extremely competitive. I vividly recall trading baseball cards with Uncle Jr., who never went easy on me. My mom always rooted for the hometown team, yelled as loudly as any fan at the TV screen, and loved being at the game. I wished she were here today, but she was watching the race on TV, hoping to catch a glimpse of me. I had no idea till the sibling rivalry between my mom and Uncle Jr. moved to a group text around mile twenty-one; I was not only racing against 49,999 other runners, but also against my uncle Jr.'s time in his own New York City Marathon from sixteen years ago. While I ran, he was tracking my pace to see if I had a chance to beat his time from 2000. And he held nothing back as he boasted to Mom about his thoughts on my chances. They verbally jabbed with a few right and left hooks before finishing with a few well-spoken uppercuts: all over text messaging. This was my mother, certain her son would beat his uncle Jr., guaranteeing she could gloat for the rest of the evening, at least.

I saw Andrea one last time at mile twenty-two. We chatted briefly, and my engine turned from classic car to modern Ferrari. She looked proud, and I wanted to impress her. I fired up and rounded the corner after the twenty-third-mile marker: Jordan-esque. I round another corner to chants of "Charles!" I assumed that it was another group of spectators reading my shirt. I ran right past my friends Mike and Cynthia. I circled back quickly, high-fived him, hugged Cynthia, and got back on the course.

The final 5K was smooth. I imagined that I had just kicked into overdrive to close out the last three miles, but in reality, it was seeing my friends and family toward the end that gave me a final burst of energy. Mentally, I kept thinking about what distance was left and not the total I'd run. Passing mile twenty-five, as I hung a right turn on Central Park South, my mind started to go bananas. It was exactly a year ago that I had been on the other side of this spectator-lined fence, watching as the runners made their final laps while gazing into the eyes of the finishers. I had lived here for ten years and had never taken that walk before. I don't know what had possessed me to do so exactly twelve months prior; maybe it had been God telling me, "You need to challenge yourself in a different way. This is the time."

When you make that final right turn heading north approaching mile twenty-six, you know you've made it. There's a row of flags on each side lining the last two hundred meters that reminds you of the global presence of the competitors. The brisk wind made the flags blow. The bleacher seats provided the final cheers to take me past the finish line. I soaked in every bit of those final moments by walking the last two-tenths of a mile because I had no clue what was going to happen next. I wanted that feeling to last as long as possible: bliss. There were runners who crawled the final stretch, to pass the blue timing strip on the ground, as names and their respective countries were called out. I too, crossed that line. Soon after, I was awarded my first marathon medal.

Here's what they don't tell you about running in November and sweating for five-plus hours (I didn't beat Uncle Jr.'s time): you'll have another mile to go before you can even get out of the barricaded areas. I was walking and now freezing in forty-degree weather. My legs, back, and arms were starting to cramp. I had prepurchased the finishers' lined poncho, which helped . . . a little. Every step I took reverberated through my bones and thighs. At that moment, the chaffing of my arms from constantly brushing past my torso and of my legs from brushing past each other crept into my mind, and I realized parts of my body were burning. If I stopped moving, though, it would only put off the opportunity to get into a shower, put on fresh clothes, and crawl into bed. I finally got out, and through a sea of runners, I saw Andrea with a bottle of champagne in her hands. She cheered and popped open the bottle. The sound of the cork pop was like the wrong music for a sentimental occasion. I felt more eager to sip tea in bed than champagne on the street.

Earlier that year, we had been in Monte Carlo for the Monaco edition of Formula 1. I had been there a few years prior while living in Italy and knew I had to come back. We watched the race from a yacht party that we had snuck into and were only a few hundred feet away from Lewis Hamilton when he was presented with the winner's trophy. Later that mid-May evening, as we were preparing to go out, I remembered I hadn't taken my vitamins that morning and figured, why not wash them down with champagne?

Andrea stared at me, puzzled. "What are you doing?"

Casually, I responded, "You know. Champagne and vitamins." As an ode to celebration and lifestyle, I secured the Instagram handle and domain name the very next day.

At this moment, I couldn't even think about champagne. I could only think about how I was going to get home from Seventieth Street and Central Park West. The traffic was crawling. Racers and spectators packed the streets like sardines.

The rideshares and Ubers were booked. And everyone held their hands up, praying for a yellow cab. We ducked into a Starbucks for a moment, and I slurped down a coffee, hoping the caffeine could somehow fix the aches in my body. It didn't.

I got home, showered, and put on fresh clothes. We went to Keens Steakhouse, one of my favorites for celebration dinners. Keens houses over fifty thousand clay pipes; it's like one for every runner. It would become my New York City Marathon tradition. I added a new title to my repertoire: marathoner.

Chapter 07

Black Men Don't Run Marathons?

In those weeks leading up to Philadelphia, it hadn't even crossed my mind to not run that race. My subconscious had already decided for me. If my conscious mind connected the events leading up to my first marathon, my subconscious integrated denouement and decided I was going to Philadelphia.

I had no clue at this point what the marathon blues were, but I know now I had it. There is no feeling quite like it: the emptiness, the rush, the joy. As you make your way into the last few miles, and then the last one, you feel like you are flying. All the discomfort and pain that may be throbbing in your joints or muscles become easy to ignore thanks to that one-of-a-kind high. Afterward, of course, there is the drop-off—the marathon blues. This is a different kind of emptiness altogether, one that is much less freeing and much more grating. What can you do?

Retired professional athletes must have it the worst—the letdown experienced as the cheering ends. I watched an interview with Sugar Ray Leonard, who endured substance abuse while attempting to relive the high of competing after he had retired. I felt a mild case of this but was buoyed by the fact that I had the Philly race coming in just two weeks. I had just run up First Avenue with a hundred thousand people yelling my name. With the crossing of the finish line, that adulation was over. I would never have another hundred thousand spectators yelling my name . . . that is, until the next race.

The streets were lined with lava. At least, the heat made it feel like it. Stairs shot arrows into my thighs, giving me intermittent claudication, a medical term for cramping pain in the leg induced by exercise. *Claudication* comes from the Latin word *claudus*, meaning "lame." Fitting, because this pain I was experiencing was so lame. The chalky light reached down from the sky and blinded me into exhaustion. I felt like one of Tyson's early opponents when he knocked them out in seconds. The fountain of marathon joy, love, and romance had already left by Tuesday. I needed a week off, not just a day. And I was about to pick up like nothing had happened the last two weeks, just to turn around and do it again.

The Philadelphia Marathon was originally a succedaneum, a winning substitute, for the failure that was bound to happen to many runners in New York City. In fact, it was well known that many New Yorkers signed up for Philly knowing that if they failed in the Big Apple and they were still capable of running, they could amend their mishap by driving ninety miles or so south to the City of Brotherly Love. So I had dropped the $130 for registration as a consolation prize should I not finish the New York City Marathon.

I have always loved Philadelphia. I moved to Manhattan in 2005 after finishing up a tumultuous time in East Lansing, Michigan. Michigan winters are cold, dark, and lonely, even if you're surrounded by family and friends. The summers are humid and daunting. I always knew I'd be leaving sooner or later. On weekends, if I had nothing to do in New York, I'd hop on the Bolt or Megabus to Philly for the day. I felt very comfortable on Broad Street. I'd have a cheesesteak, visit The Philadelphia Museum of Art, walk around the city for a few hours, and catch the last bus home. I repeated this numerous times until I moved to Rome in 2009.

The start of the Philly race seemed normal. After finishing New York City just two weeks prior, I was certain this would be a breeze. Besides, I was playing with house money at this point; I had nothing to lose. They couldn't take back my first medal. I strolled up to the starting line like an experienced quarterback ready to take the final snap in a lopsided game I was winning. I had not announced this race on my social media because, well, I wasn't really planning to run today anyway. There was no group of friends waiting along the course, and the only people I expected to see were Andrea and Arline. The cheers were silenced by the name missing from the front of my shirt. No one was yelling, "Go, Charles!" I could bow out of this race with relatively few people knowing I had even started it.

I was six or seven miles into the race when I started to notice something anomalous. In New York City, the course goes through all five boroughs, and unless you turn around, you're constantly facing the back of your fellow runners ahead of you. In Philly, the out and backs allow you to see the runners' faces in a way that was not present in Manhattan. When I saw other

Black runners, they noticed me and interacted first. They always acknowledged me with a nod of their heads.

I knew what that meant. I have often been in a room where we as a racial group were in the few. It could be elite educational institutions, event spaces, restaurants, or other places, but I knew that nod. I wondered why they were giving it to me. I originally thought it was because it was the City of Brotherly Love. But it wasn't everyone. It was only my brothers, my Black brothers. I tucked that thought into the back of my mind to ponder more during the second half of the race.

I went into research mode after the marathon. I had Monday free for the second time. I stayed home on the computer to research Black people and marathons while starting the documentary *Marathon: The Patriots Day Bombing*. I found an article with a short phrase: "Black people don't run marathons." It provided some statistics, perspectives, and reasons why media figure Marcus Ryder felt marathoning was a White, elitist sport. This launched me down a rabbit hole. An article in *Runner's World* asked, "Why Is Running So White?" I had no clue this was a thing.

I researched marathons to understand why they were considered elitist. I thought that a pair of sneakers, some gym shorts, and a T-shirt was all you needed, but I was beginning to understand that marathon history was deeper than that. Running was always marketed to middle- and upper-class White people. Nike pitched their shoes for jogging as a leisure sport to increase general health. Running, then marathoning, was sold with the shoes as the center. Whites had a head start. These options were not pitched to Blacks. Middle- and upper-class Blacks did not feel safe running in their White neighborhoods. Running clubs were all White for that reason. Then I started to consider the race registration fees and all the gear pitched at the expos. Let's not get started with traveling, airline tickets, hotel lodging fees, and restaurant bills. My head started spinning, so I went back to the documentary about the Boston Marathon bombing. Yeah, 'cause that'll be more uplifting . . . not.

Chapter 08

Warrior Mode!

I now had roughly six weeks to prepare for a marathon in Orlando, Florida, which meant I was running between three and five miles per day, two to three times per week. My undertraining continued, but so did my drive to finish. I slightly adjusted my diet. I have always been a healthy eater, but now carbohydrates became a positive. The constant movement burned through them like fossil fuels in a West Virginia government building. Issues that plague African Americans at record percentages, like diabetes, wouldn't play out in my purposeful carb-loading . . . I hoped. Carb-loading the week of the race was par for the course.

Hydration was also a new word in my vocabulary. It's true that we are all different, but I sweat when I feel pressure, and when the temperature is above sixty-five, just thinking about sweating makes me sweat. In other words, hydration-related cramps, or hyponatremia, was constantly top of mind for me. I also hammered out a plan to maintain my sodium levels during races so that issues like fatigue, nausea, and headaches would not affect me on race day. It's all about balance.

I was at an emotional low going into the new year and my third marathon. What should've been joyous was kind of miserable. I felt a little unsure of what I was doing and why I was running another marathon. My crying over the bombing had ceased, but the heartfelt intensity I had felt from watching the tragedies of *Marathon: The Patriots Day Bombing* was heightened by the fact I actually ran marathons. I still wanted to know why those brothers had so much evil inside them and why a system would be put in place to make marathoning an accomplishment reserved for a select group of people. To top it off, my friends were questioning my choices for health reasons. Questions about my knees and joints and heart had started entering my conversations. And I wondered if I'd still have gotten those questions if I was approaching age twenty-one as opposed to forty-one.

In a single moment, the temptation can become irresistible to just go with the flow, play it by ear, wing it. We have all done it, and to confuse matters further, some have succeeded in doing it at some point too. When that happens, it reinforces all our worst mindsets and habits, convincing us that if we show up, even without any plan, it will all work out.

I had trained myself to believe I didn't have to plan, to believe that nothing could ever go wrong. Call it confidence, or maybe a little bit of arrogance. Of course, things *can* go wrong. One small error can turn into a bigger oversight, which can turn into a short-term issue, which can build into a long-term problem. You learn too late that, more often than not, not planning is a costly risk.

There is an old saying that describes this: if you fail to plan, then you plan to fail. One decision leads to the next. Unless you know what you're doing and you have taken the time to pinpoint and prepare for all that can go awry, you are just asking for trouble. By failing to plan, you may as well plan to slip into crisis. Sooner or later, tragedy will strike, and without a strategy, you won't know how to get out of it.

This is true for any fitness goal. Those who wing it and succeed are often simply lucky. All other success stories come from planning because, as unglamorous as planning may be, it is the one thing that stands between you and every worst-case scenario your instincts tell you to ignore.

With my running, I didn't just want to prove something to myself. I still don't quite know why I planned on doing something this nuts, but I have my suspicions. I was very emotional after the Philadelphia Marathon. The bombing was a big reason, but the lopsided inclusion statistics really lit a fire inside of me. I wanted to set an example for Black men and women. I had no clue if it would ignite anything in anyone, but showing, instead of telling, was the only way I knew how. And I felt I needed to go on a journey to show that Black people ran marathons, from city to city, across the globe. My plan was to run twelve marathons between November 2016 and November 2017. I mapped out the cities:

November 2016: New York City, New York and Philadelphia, Pennsylvania
January 2017: Orlando, Florida
February 2017: Birmingham, Alabama
March 2017: Washington, DC

April 2017: Rome, Italy and Boston, Massachusetts
May 2017: Pittsburgh, Pennsylvania
Summer: off
September 2017: Berlin, Germany
October 2017: Chicago, Illinois, and Washington, DC
November 2017: New York City, New York and Philadelphia,
Pennsylvania

I can't really explain the ebullience of going to Orlando. It
wasn't a major marathon city ... or so I thought. Maybe it was the
kid in me returning to Disney World for the first time since I was
seven. My sister, Hazel, and I were the only ones born at that time,
and being only two years apart, we had torn through the park
like Bonnie and Clyde (which is the nickname my Aunt Debbie
had given us). We took a rocket ship ride to Mars at EPCOT,
skipped through Cinderella Castle at the Magic Kingdom, and
spent a year's allowance at every gift shop within our grasp: we
loved Mickey and Minnie.

It was early January, and the air was crisp in New York
City. The Uber arrived on time, so I made my 9 a.m. flight out
of LaGuardia Airport, and it didn't smell like old motor oil and
dried puke from last night's drunk passengers. You know, the
usual. The airport was without lines, and it was a good thing;
Andrea hates airport lines. Everything was clicking. Like a bald
eagle, I was flying south for the winter, and the plane ride was as
smooth as a quantum-stabilized atom mirror. Yeah, *that* smooth.
But when we were disembarking from the airplane cabin, I
realized I had misfired on my attire. Since when had Disney
become a giant industrial freezer? I was in shorts, and it was two
degrees below freezing. "Here goes my first race in Antarctica,"
I mumbled.

The Walt Disney World Marathon is a real weekend affair. Grown men and women come from all over the country, dressed in their best impressions of Mickey, Minnie, Goofy, and Donald. Halloween is usually in October—but not to the folks running at Disney. First, this is one of the few marathons not included in the Abbott World Marathon Majors list of six events where you need to pay off the door guy to get in. If you complete the entire four-part series during the Walt Disney World Marathon Weekend races on pace, you earn four individual event medals, Goofy's Race and a Half Challenge medal, and the Dopey Challenge medal. All in all, it's a bit more than forty-eight miles and nearly $700 in registration fees alone. I called my banker. My loan was denied, and Walt's guy Bob Iger rejected my firstborn; I settled for just Sunday's marathon.

It was Disney, but I was entering warrior mode. The gear upgrade was significant. It was no longer just a marathon. I was going to war, reviving Simba's battle for Pride Rock. First things first: I tossed aside my ASICS GEL-NIMBUS 18s for HOKA Bondis. It was a small weight increase, with significantly more cushion. I thought about protecting my joints and didn't want to spend my future cogitating or mispronouncing words like *acetabulum* and *hemiarthroplasty*. (Try pronouncing those two aloud after three glasses of wine.) I also started a new ritual of taping my ankles, knees, and hips. KT Tape—or kinesiology therapeutic tape, for those mere mortals who never get injured—is elastic sports tape designed to provide drug-free pain relief or muscle support. I taped my ankles, calves, shins, full knees, and hips. Of course, I had to watch a YouTube video like sixteen times to get it right since this was my first time using it. So far, I had no aches or pains, and research told me that heavier shoes and tape would slow me down. But my concern was taking care of my body rather than improving my time.

I presented my goal to myself in my head while at the expo like a professor preparing for a grand lecture: *I am running twelve marathons from November 2016 to November 2017,* I repeated over and over in my head. I was not kidding myself. Jordan retired when he was forty. I was beginning my athletic career at forty. This was no longer a bucket list about one race or cashing in on a contingency plan. This was now a mission. I had not talked about myself as a marathoner up to this point. My friends had seen me in that way before I had. The shift didn't occur within me, but as the integration of a marathoner persona into my daily lifestyle. The consummate undertrainer became the example of fitness and nutrition. But I still only trained on a treadmill and ran outside only when there was a sanctioned race. I was not only defiant against the people who thought I could not compete; I was committed to the mission. I was not saying it aloud as a mere boast. I felt that I would embody the Black man running marathons to whoever was watching. Everyone who sees me knows I am Black. What I was doing was the ultimate revocation of the veil of elitism.

"And I'm not even a runner," I said over and over.

I'm hubristic one moment, then I seek attention by telling you what I'm not or incapable of doing so. Like over and over claiming I'm *not* a runner—even at this point. Andrea loves correcting me whenever given the opportunity. She swiftly replied, "You just ran a couple of half-marathons, a Spartan trifecta, and two marathons back-to-back. You can't say you're not a runner anymore."

The race started at five-thirty in the morning. I imagine the good folks at Disney World wanted to get us in and out of their parks as soon as possible to minimally interrupt their usual family-friendly follies. Not even a trap set by Scar could stop me from waking up and running this race. But buyer beware: it was like being lost in the labyrinth designed by a deranged white rabbit (your faulty map), and even your morning magical potion (a sports drink) won't help you to the starting line. I exited the hotel and was already late for the shuttle ride. I was told there was another one about a half mile down leaving a different property. I missed that one too. The Uber app was useless. Luckily, I found a guy snoring in his jitney cab, and I always keep $40 on me for emergencies during every race. Lions aren't the only kings ... so is cash.

"Excuse me, sir. I'm trying to reach the starting line of the Disney marathon. Can you help?"

He responded swiftly, "Sure, that'll cost you ..."

I panicked. "Will two twenties do it?"

My eyes were still glued together from the lack of sleep. If he took me to Miami, I probably wouldn't realize it until maybe we encountered the Three Lakes Wildlife Management Area, where I might be awakened by the begging call of some brown pelicans. He took winding roads leading to the starting line with the same fierceness of those birds. We arrived, and on time. And I was short two Jacksons.

Disney would be my first encounter with race fanatics. I started to notice them right away. Certain marathons have their fans. At this point, I still did not understand why. People have lists of accomplishments they are concerned with. It may be the majors, completion times, or something else. My initial desire to run was to achieve the New York City Marathon runners' look of exhausted accomplishment as they crossed the finish line.

Here, at every mile marker was a Disney character. And this clued me in as to why Disney has one of the longest cutoff times for when the last runner's time would officially count. (Runners must maintain a sixteen-minute-mile pace.) Lines of adults in costumes waited patiently to grab a selfie or portrait with the carefree Mickey, the elegant Cinderella, the boastful Peter Pan, or next to the jovial veneer of Stromboli. It didn't matter the size of the line, only that they ended with twenty-six photos. Disney marathon runners are maniacs.

The race starts at Epcot Center. Epcot opened in 1982, and my parents first took me and Hazel just two years later. We would then pass through the original theme park, the Magic Kingdom, and see Cinderella Castle on Main Street. It's impressive how pristine they kept the Disney grounds, as if the seven dwarfs scrubbed every inch of the pavement after every visitor walked by. Then came the African savanna-inspired Animal Kingdom. It looked so real I kept my guard up just in case I had to dodge an errant laughing hyena. It never came. The Hollywood Studios and the ESPN Wide World of Sports Complex were both a letdown. It lacked the vigor and childlike experience of the other parks, but we ended with a revisit to Epcot, which made me think of how excited Hazel and I had been when we had returned to Detroit to show off our souvenir loot as kids, feeling less like Peter Pan and more like Captain Hook.

I made it. This would be my third marathon in as many months. I crossed the finish line and gave a sigh of relief. All the joy in the air, watching the racers stop for selfies with Disney characters, seemed a good distraction at each mile marker. The KT Tape made my legs stiff, but injuries were not in the cards. I felt like this race was about tests. I was testing out safety measures and wanted to make sure I would be safe, even in this bubble of a racecourse. I popped over to a store and bought a set of Mickey Mouse ears and took a picture in front of the Hulk. Although Run Disney was fun; I felt powerful.

The flight back home was more eventful than I had thought it would be. We were waiting to board, and something felt off. Andrea approached the desk at the flight gate, and they informed her that, due to overbooking, they were asking for six passengers to take a later flight to accommodate a family from London who needed to make a connection in Atlanta. You've got to love Delta Airlines. They offered any willing soul a $500 credit to get put up in a two-star hotel around the corner and be shuttled back the next morning for a new flight. Andrea and I agreed that we would be two of those willing souls. We just needed four more to make our triumphant march to the shuttle. Otherwise, the deal was off.

We waited. And waited. They upped the pot of gold. And finally, two more characters popped up: Cathy and her boyfriend. Cathy had been running marathons for years, and she was an adult who loved Disney. A native New Yorker and an experienced traveler, she drooled over where she could go with the extra $800. I noticed Cathy's medal.

"How was your race?" I asked with curiosity.

Cathy was so excited about this crazy feat she'd accomplished. "I did the Dopey Challenge. I'm exhausted," she panted.

We began to chat about her race career and exchanged notes for about an hour. The pot was up to $1,200 per person. I crossed my fingers that some poverty-stricken passenger would renounce their love for riding thirty thousand feet in the air again and take the bait. Their golden voices instructed us where to find our chariot, they handed us our winnings, and within the hour, we were eating pizza out of a cardboard box before bed.

Cathy was the first friend I made in the marathon community. She was a vet. She had already run over five marathons, trained indoors and outdoors, and was a woman with a plan. Over the next couple of years, we met during shorter races, running side by side at 5Ks and 10Ks, and grabbing a coffee after other races. We remain friends today, often texting about training, races, and ways to stay motivated. I learned the value of community. You seek out a tribe wherever you go. I was not running with a club, so I did not have a ready-made community. I only ran outside on race day, so I was not engaged with others. My races were individual. They were *my* races. Though people were all around, they were running their own races too. In later years, I would expand my marathon community. The significance of this was tangible. It extends beyond just sharing gear, experiences, successes, and challenges centered on the common practice of running marathons.

I also learned the importance of patience. I was in a constant space of learning. After Orlando, I finally thought of myself as a marathoner. I no longer harbored any imposter syndrome inside me. I was not the typical runner who had begun in high school or college. I had begun at forty. Every time I would tell someone about the marathons, they would remind me of my age: "Did you run track or cross-country in high school or college?" "Were you always a runner?" I'd get these questions all the time, and it would feel like an interrogation. That feeling slowly started to subside as my confidence ascended alongside my experience. Marathoners peaked at thirty-seven. I was already forty, and I had so much more to accomplish. There were nine more marathons on the calendar for the remainder of the year, and I had no reason to think I wouldn't be bringing home nine more medals. I was here to prove them wrong. This warrior was ready for another battle.

Chapter 09

Time for Silence.

Our greatest hopes are shaped by the environment we are raised in. I'd love to say the deeply rooted African American history of Birmingham, Alabama, is what brought me to the Deep South, but it was actually the title sponsor: Mercedes-Benz. Growing up in Detroit, a city that birthed American luxury vehicles such as Cadillac and Lincoln, we still admire the craftsmanship of the Benz and the Beamer. The car meant more than just style; Mercedes was a status symbol. Right or wrong, it's an idiosyncrasy familiar to many of us; it's a kind of toy that can lead the people around you to assume you're a certain kind of person or that you've made it. The finisher's medal you receive at the Mercedes-Benz Marathon race is just like the emblem emblazoned on the front of their iconic vehicles.

Up until this point, the cities I chose were considered cool. Unfortunately, in Andrea's opinion, Birmingham, Alabama, missed the cut. She couldn't care less about the medal and had no interest in hanging out there. "I'll see you when you return," she said in a flat and unexcited tone that stung a little. I often traveled alone, but there was something comforting about having a partner during a marathon weekend in case I got injured, ended up sick, or just flat-out DNF a big race.

Am I being vacuous? I asked myself, followed by, *Why am I really going there?* Her tone made me rethink my actions. *I'm going to get in, get my Benz emblem, and get out,* I thought to myself.

One night a few days before the race, I was flipping through the documentary section on HBO. I came across the 1997 Spike Lee joint, *4 Little Girls*, a film about the murder of four African American girls in the 1963 bombing of the Sixteenth Street Baptist Church in Birmingham. I pushed Play.

The Baptist Church bombing goes down in the history books as merely a perpetuation of racial segregation. Located on Sixteenth Street, only blocks from where I would be staying, the church was bombed on Sunday, September 15, 1963, killing four girls and injuring dozens of others. In the year leading up to the bombing, Birmingham was tense and violent toward Blacks. The situation was so volatile that racial integration of any form was met with violent resistance. Once again, a documentary centered on an act of domestic terrorism had me in tears leading up to a race.

Watching this moment in time was like reading current headlines in *The New York Times* or any other American newspaper: a stark reminder that not much has changed when it comes to diversity, equity, inclusion and, in general, humanity. I sat on my sofa contemplating my reasons for going to Birmingham and whether I wanted to take part in this race at all. I told myself I had to be there. It was no longer just about the marathon—it was about the people in this city.

When I finally arrived in Birmingham on the Saturday morning of the race, I hailed a taxi from the airport with the confidence of a local.

Upon rolling down his window, the cabby asked, "Where do you want to go?" with a furrowed brow, indicating that if I stated the wrong location, he would politely move on to the next customer.

"I'm here to see the church where the four girls were murdered and the civil rights museum," I responded with the firmness of a chain-link fence.

He unlocked the doors, I tossed my duffel bag into the back seat, and off we went.

I skipped mentioning the marathon because at that moment, it didn't matter as long I made it to the expo before 5 p.m. My mission was cultural, and the marathon didn't matter. We pulled up to Sixth Avenue North and Sixteenth Street North, stopping just east of the church. His eyes led me to believe that he saw the pain in mine.

"Take as long as you want. I'm stopping the meter," the driver muttered with a southern drawl that sounded straight out of the film *Driving Miss Daisy*.

I realized why Birmingham was culturally important for me to visit. I had to see the sculpture of *The Four Spirits*. I needed to see the four little girls' names—Addie Mae Collins, Cynthia Wesley, Carole Robertson, and Carol Denise McNair—etched in stone. I walked around the bronze memorial and felt the loss of their lives enter my spirit, the conduit being the presence of their legacy in the air. I lost myself. I stared at them for over an hour before returning to the vehicle. We remained silent as we drove to the museum.

The Birmingham Civil Rights Institute is a modern museum established in 1992 to document the activities and major milestones of local civil rights movements, all of which were pivotal in the fight for human rights in the United States. The museum exhibits activists' and Alabama residents' struggles and sacrifices during the 1950s and 1960s Civil Rights Movements. Historically, such movements in the United States, especially prior to the 1970s, were violently opposed by White supremacy groups and racially biased police officers. The museum commemorates these struggles that aimed to change our American society for the better.

I felt it heightened the emotions I had experienced at the church. It felt so real seeing the memorial and the museum back-to-back. The intimacy of these experiences was visceral. As I walked through the galleries, I read stories, saw images, and watched the emotions of other visitors as we were reminded of the way Black Americans were treated by their community at large. I wish I had blown through the museum like I was going to speed through the marathon tomorrow, taking no prisoners and wasting no time. But I couldn't help but slowly take it all in, and then my generous driver was awaiting to take me to my hotel.

The marathon itself was rather eventless. This city, in all its history, didn't move me. I was still processing the feelings and experiences I had had the day before, and I could think of nothing else. The racecourse comprised two revolutions around one big circle. I felt like Phil Connors running around to see the chubby rodent in *Groundhog Day*.

I returned home the Sunday evening after the marathon and thought about the lives lost during those tragic years in states like Alabama. The only thing I'd lost in Birmingham was my toenail. Hematoma (a swelling of clotted blood) occurs so frequently for endurance athletes and marathoners that it's almost like a badge of honor. For me, it was the most disgusting thing that I'd ever experienced. If you're lucky enough to have healthy blood clotting on your scars, you might accumulate that same flow of water, salt, protein, and cells underneath an area receiving constant pounding, like that spot underneath the nail plate. While running, the toes are slamming against your shoe, creating sort of a microtrauma, and the more you run, the more you subject your feet to this traumatic experience.

Thinking about this, I thought to myself, *Do they still add up if you only run outside on race day?* Apparently, if you're running, you run the risk of losing a toenail no matter where you plant your feet.

My post-race routine was somber. That Monday, I lay around the house, feeling like I was searching for answers. I thought about Cathy, my new friend whom I had met in Orlando. While volunteering for an NYRR race, I met a guy named Matt. Matt was thirtysomething, Jewish, and a native New Yorker who made a living designing some of the advertisements that caught the eye of the cool millennials. He did work for adidas and other major brands. He was a fast talker and ran even faster. I was slowly building up my personal community of friends who run. Cathy had stories for days about ruining toenails, so she just laughed it off. "It'll grow back," she muttered.

"Bro, just wait till you're on the sideline with a real injury," Matt spit back at me.

But I also contemplated some numbers in Birmingham. The city is 70 percent Black or African American. Yet the marathon

demographics in the city didn't come close to matching that
number. Why didn't more Black people run marathons?
I contemplated and theorized about the rationale for this
disparity. Do we fear losing our toenails? Or were marathons
secretly planned on Sundays as part of some master plan to
hide from unsuspecting groups? That would be some creative
systemic racism. Marathoning is painful. Maybe we in the Black
community suffer from algophobia, or a fear of pain.

By the time of the Birmingham race, the only Black marathoner
I knew personally was my uncle Jr. A couple of my Black friends
were athletic, some a couple of years younger, and even played
organized sports at some point in their lives. They ran, but they
weren't runners. Their goals were different. Many of them knew
what a marathon was, but often lamented, "That's stuff that White
people do." I had no clue that was a thing. I was as oblivious to
this way of thinking just like Alicia Silverstone might be about
the medicinal benefits of castor oil or swag surfin'. "That's stuff
that Black people do." I just followed what my mind, body, and
spirit told me to do.

It was clear I was an athlete-masochist. All these things
crossed my mind except my missing toenail as I tried not to think
about it. It hurt like hell. Taking care of the feet made its way into
my Google searches. I read about Mebrahtom "Meb" Keflezighi,
an Ethiopian-born champion, who runs under the American
flag. Many marathon winners are Kenyan or Ethiopian. On the
elite scale, they often place in the top ten and break records.
Keflezighi talks candidly about his injuries.

At this time, in my mind, safety and protection centered
on my knees. Whenever I'd talk about marathoning, some
concerned citizen would respond, "Aren't you concerned about

your knees?" No one ever asked about spiked cortisol levels or reactive oxygen species. Hyponatremia? Or my biggest concern— all the air pollution I was sucking up. If they knew anything about running, they'd be asking about my toes. Or maybe about safety for my life, *running while Black*, during training.

Still, I purchased the best (or at least, the most expensive) running shoes: HOKA. I trusted that as long as I spent at least $180 on sneakers, all would be okay. My toenail was bruised and resembled a nasty-looking kaleidoscope-like mix of black and blue. But after a week, it was gone. Not the coloring . . . the actual toenail. I was shocked and slightly discouraged. It was an ugly mess. I was uncertain about what would come next. The only thing that could possibly stop me from running the next eight marathons was an injury. This was my first. The worry centered on whether it would affect my next run—which was only a few weeks away.

My own tragedy was not nearly as important, but an eerie parallel to the sense of loss and the definitions of self that resulted. The circumstances of losing the toenail were critical, along with my emotional state: time and loss became the center of gravity. How much time do we have left here? How damaging will losses be on productivity in the future? Taking the time to process the experience was critical to how I set my priorities. I had never thought I would travel to Birmingham, but I would have stayed longer if I had it to do over again. There was so much history to see there, and I had only scraped the surface.

Eventually, the toenail grew back, and I was able to rebound. In comparison, no one recovers from a tragedy; rather, as a result, they can grow and heal to varying degrees. Cultivating resilience means to radically accept the trauma and move forward anyway. The quote "Everything is happening for me and not to me" comes to mind. The toenail was a metaphor for the losses that the community of Birmingham had endured for decades. Their resilience shone, while mine seemed exaggerated. It demonstrated to me that resilience in the face of adversity, trauma, or loss takes place in a series of small moments and choices.

My experience was rich in many ways. Birmingham is a place of deep history and a living master class in resilience. I had no friends or family in attendance, but the thoughts of being there and the time I spent learning about the past are what carried me. My little brother, a walking encyclopedia when it comes to Black American history, would've loved seeing the museums and feeling the vibe of the people. It reminded me of how important family is to experiences we have in life.

Chapter 10

Friends help you get through any of life's marathons.

Who knew the Obamas wouldn't remain in Washington, DC, for another term? So Michelle decided not to run for office, and I'm running a marathon there just as the new guy was taking over. I listened to Miles Davis's *Bitches Brew* on the train ride from New York City on repeat. Arguably the greatest jazz album of all time, it was a seminal force that still impacts a new generation, not unlike those eight years we were in power in the Oval Office. Politics never excited me, but my community always did. I knew I'd see my friends from Rome. Alessandro and Caron had remained in Italy. Travis had returned to New York City. And Michael, Max, and Ryan had relocated to the capital.

^^^

My time in Rome was supposed to last only a summer.

When I was an undergrad, I was fascinated with languages and Italian culture. I applied to teach English in Messina, Sicily, in the summer of 1999. I always regretted being afraid to move to Sicily; I could've already taken a tour of the Church of the Santissima Annunziata dei Catalani, go for a boat ride on Lago di Ganzirri, or have an espresso in Zona Falcata. I promised myself that, when the opportunity presented itself again, I'd jump on it. Ten years later, I'd be starting my MBA at St. John's University, then I'd be running to the Italian consulate to secure a summer student visa. Clearly, a summer wasn't going to be enough time for me to gain a cultural understanding of Italy along with learning Italian fluently.

My summer partner in crime was Michael. He was short and thin with a southern drawl that could charm a cobra in Thailand. "What did one tectonic plate say when he bumped into the other?" Michael would joke, then finished before you'd answer, "My fault." He was our resident science nerd. He was in Rome getting a masters in international political science.

Alessandro, tall and stocky, slicked his hair back and carried himself as a proud Northern Italian. He prided himself on his diverse group of friends from all over the globe and became an honorary member of the St. John's University crew. He was the only Italian among us. Max, a Cameroonian-born polyglot who spent time in France and Germany before landing in Rome, eventually found his way to DC. Caron, a blonde and blue-eyed DC-/Maryland-/Virginia-area native, founded CMC World Travel and would remain in Italy. Queens, New York, kid Travis found himself in Rome pitching wealthy boarding-school Italians the American dream. (Italy's longest-serving prime minister, Silvio Berlusconi, even sent his daughter to St. John's.)

The summer sun would eventually fade, and I would spend the next two years living in Rome and traveling all over Europe. Italy was a lesson in art, language, architecture, food and, most importantly, wine. Along with finishing my MBA, I worked for an Italian bank after learning to speak Italian fluently. I became an expert in Italian wine, taking a world-renowned sommelier course at the Michelin triple-starred La Pergola restaurant. It was an eighteen-month intensive exercise in Italian. I continued on to fine coffee, becoming a regular at Il Piccolo Diavolo in the Prati zone and Il Cigno in Parioli. A kid named Ryan would take Michael's place once Michael returned to America. One by one, small groups of going-away parties would see off the rest of the crew, leaving me to realize that my own time would soon end. The end of 2011 would be the end of an era. Each person's departure felt like a series of mini-reunions.

When I think of the time I spent in Rome, my most vivid memories are when we were all together as a group. This scene would play out again in Washington, DC.

^^^

It was cold and damp. The air was so thick it was like you were swimming in Lambert's Cove—in off-peak season. The juxtaposition of the weather from Birmingham to DC mimicked the political climate at this time: icy hot. We recently had had the changing of the guard. But all I could think about was changing my clothes. I woke up with the haste of being late for my own birthday party. Following the general rule of marathons on Sunday, the race would be starting in minutes, and I was still taping my body parts.

I arrived near Constitution Avenue Northwest and Fourteenth Street Southwest on the National Mall at the starting line, but no one was there. Confused, I approached a twentysomething woman and asked, "Where exactly is the starting line of the marathon?"

The young woman looked as if she was trying to stifle laughter as she answered, "I'm sorry, sir. The last runner crossed the starting line over twenty minutes ago." It was almost as if she had been rehearsing this speech just for me all morning. She said it so casually and without any regard for my race bib, which clearly stated I was supposed to be in the race.

Usually, the ticking of a clock means boredom, the passage of time, or it means progress, being in time. Running late, however, one realizes all too well—painfully so—the other significance that the ticking of a clock can take on. You may not be able to participate!

From your fingertips, more tingly now than they were a moment before, to your heartbeat, racing swiftly to some unknown destination, the anxiety creeps in, nestling snugly in the part of your mind that knows time can't go backward and yet still insists on wishing it would. Running late, one has one solution: get there, beat the clock, and make the clock's ticking boring once again. I was sensing the impending danger of missing the race and hoping the gods (that is, the race organizers) weren't keeping score.

Races are timed and scores are kept. Each runner has some type of timing chip, either embedded on the back of the race bib or in the form of a tiny device you might clip on your shoelace. Either way, it's supplied to ensure that your race time is attached to the person who registered for the race. The chip is activated once you cross a timing strip at the start of the event, and the peroration at the end gives your final race time. Larger races have checkpoints throughout the course to help runners understand their inter-race pacing. One must cross the start and finish lines for the race to count. I looked around for the start strip, ignoring her warnings that it was too late.

I looked all over, my once discombobulated face now wearing the not-so-subtle hint of resoluteness. "You'll have to first catch me, then tackle me!" I yelled. My voice faded as I burst over the starting strip like a volcanic eruption from Mount Tambora. And for the next thirty seconds, even Usain Bolt couldn't have caught me.

As I drove my feet into the ground, the adrenaline warmed my body, my blood circulating rapidly and the carbohydrate metabolism amping me up. If you had extracted it from my body, you could have fueled a Ferrari F12berlinetta. I ran. And I ran. I was at war with the back end of the race. *Guerra*, the Italian word for *war*, came to mind because I knew I'd be seeing my friends from Rome once I got through this grueling endeavor.

I had never seen the end of the line before. I started to hear music coming from up ahead. I'd hoped I'd be approaching racers, but it was merely beats from the first band. At every mile marker, there was a band of some sort, banging on drums, yelling into a microphone, or plucking strings. I remembered the Alamo. My destiny was starting to manifest. I would not be last. As I passed the sweepers, including the lady carrying a balloon that designated the pace for the last official finisher, I knew I was gaining ground on my friendly foes. I blocked out the music with the drums of my own playlist. I needed control of my environment. It took passing a couple of hundred runners before I settled into the race. I slowed my pace because there was no way I was going to maintain a 731 horsepower speed.

After I'd settled down to more like 23 horsepower at around the fourth-mile marker, I started wondering, *Why isn't there a hip-hop marathon series?*

The Rock 'n' Roll Running Series is a group of marathons that are run all over the world. Like Disney, the Rock 'n' Roll series has its audience. They target marathon runners who happen to also be fans of rock music: another niche audience that is strikingly White-dominated. I'm daydreaming about hearing a band cover "So Fresh, So Clean" while I'm sweating profusely as I'm running the Atlanta marathon. Or blasting Ice Cube, Dr. Dre, and Snoop Dogg, keeping a steady tempo on the 405 and setting a new personal record. Maybe Black people would run more marathons if we had organizations catering to our cultural desires.

I wouldn't break my personal record that race. In fact, this would become my worst time to date, as I would finish one minute slower than my first marathon. I came out too hot.

^^^

I hadn't seen the boys since Michael's wedding last year. Suddenly, the marathon didn't mean a thing. I walked in to see Max, Michael, and Ryan with smiles plastered on all their faces. Our last reunion had been in Charleston, South Carolina, all dressed up in matching tuxedos, welcoming the matrimony of Michael and Lauren. But here we stood, relaxed, catching up. It felt like Rome all over again, but without the baroque Bernini sculpted fountain and Pope Benedict XIII-inaugurated steps of

Piazza di Spagna as our backdrop. We never mentioned a word about the 26.2 miles I had just run. We talked about our families, our jobs, our recent travels, and the last time we had spoken to Alessandro, Travis, or Caron. Our friendship was bigger than any race or event.

We all want to bask in the joy and pride that comes with achievement. You pat yourself on the back, you repeat some positive affirmations, and you even buy yourself a treat just so you know you're celebrating. But all that work, thought, and effort will amount to almost nothing at all when compared with the support that you get from your people.

Among your tribe, you feel the true rush of accomplishment. It isn't in your head, but in their applause and the adoration of your community. They let you know you have made it. In their smiles, not your own, you find the fullness of all you have done. The joy and pride become real, more tangible, when you can see them outside of yourself.

The real friends. During the challenging and life-changing times, they were there. Because they saw you through, you promised yourself you would remember. You would keep them in your heart, cherishing all the energy they bestowed upon you. There is the crux of the matter: Without them, the accomplishment may have been too much for you, and with them, it never would be. Friends help you get through any of life's marathons.

To find yourself, start seeing all the incredible souls who are trying to find you too. You belong together; a single, cohesive unit, bearing life's pains together so that, when you come through the other side, you can devour life's rewards together.

Chapter 11

Ciao Roma!

R ome just might be the most beautiful city in the world. It looks a lot like any other European city; it's certainly much older than the ones in the United States. This ancient metropolis is more compact and richer with the dirt of millennia stuck on the feet of citizens and tourists alike, tracked through the paved or cobblestone streets. Of course, as anyone who has visited Rome can tell you, it is unique among even the most illustrious cities on the continent. This is not only because of the history—history is, in Europe, not scarce. If you want it, you can find it. Rome is unique, though, because of something much rarer: its captivating beauty.

Let's start in Vatican City, situated in the northwest center of Rome. Here, the popes have celebrated mass at the mammoth Basilica of St. Peter for hundreds of years. They have blessed Christian pilgrims venturing into the Holy City to hear a homily and to see the luxury with which the church decorated its homeland. The smallest country on the planet, Vatican City is home to some of the most striking pieces to survive the Renaissance, from statues to paintings. One can wander this place and never run out of sights to see, landmarks researched online and then experienced in person.

Chief among these landmarks in Vatican City is the Sistine Chapel. It was here that Michelangelo envisioned the Holy Bible and commemorated his faith. For four years in the sixteenth century, the master lay on a platform, covering the ceiling in images that would forever shape Western culture. These paintings are part of our global heritage, and until you look up and see them, you can't truly begin to know them. You can only feel the Sistine Chapel one way—with your head cocked backward, as if the clouds above had parted and the divine had appeared right then and there.

Outside Vatican City's walls, it becomes clear that the beauty found in the Basilica of St. Peter and the Sistine Chapel extends in every direction. That same beauty is in the Spanish Steps, a place I'd pass daily for Italian lessons when I lived in Rome. They loom up in breathtaking size and angle, serving as a centerpiece that connects the French-funded Trinità dei Monti Church, the Embassy of Spain, and the Holy See.

Like the Spanish Steps, the Piazza del Popolo, named for the nearby poplar trees, is at once practical and illuminating. Once the ground for public executions under the Italian monarchy, history and artistry mesh in this place as they do throughout all of Rome. No longer a place for capital punishment, it is in vogue for tourists who want a snap in front of the Egyptian obelisk of Seti I and one of the many fountains, or to brunch at the famed Hotel de Russie.

The Trevi Fountain, designed by Nicola Salvi and constructed by Giuseppe Pannini in the eighteenth century, has earned a place among all these most memorable Roman destinations. Over the centuries, it has won constant acclaim as both one of the most awe-inspiring fountains and one of the most important examples of Baroque architecture.

At the height of the Roman Empire, there was a common saying among the villagers in present-day France, Spain, and Portugal: all roads lead to Rome. In Rome, similarly, all roads lead to the artful beauty for which people all over the world cherish the city. And I was about to run 26.2 miles of those streets. How wonderful.

I had always felt at home in Rome. I remember touching down in early June 2009, taking a nap, waking up, and walking the streets until 4 a.m. I would do this over and over for the next two and a half years. The city is an urban paradise with a history of kings and emperors and notorious prime ministers. When I returned in April 2017, I felt like one of those important figures.

Andrea and I were staying a week at the home of Caron and Mauro, and she wouldn't take no for an answer to anything. It started at the airport where she sent a driver, one of her employees, to pick us up. I front-loaded the trip, so I had around a week before the marathon to get settled in, visit my old stomping grounds, hopefully see some old friends, and put my University of Siena, B2-level Italian certification back into practical use.

When I had met Caron back in 2009, she had already lived there for a decade. She had left a long career as an executive at a travel company and started CMC World Travel. By 2017, it wasn't the small outfit I had known. After a forty-five-minute drive from Fiumicino Airport, I was about to see the fruits of her empire. We arrived at the villa in Riano, just fifteen minutes or so outside of the Rome city limits: a gated, spacious home with five cars and two vans parked in the driveway.

"First things first," Caron said. "Here are the keys to your car for the week. I know you didn't think I'd be chauffeuring you around town."

Caron has always acted like the big sister I never had. She even tells everyone she's my big sister. Never mind the blonde hair and capri blue eyes—we are brother and sister. The fact was that, after being away for ten years, I was lucky to have someone treating me like any of *De vita Caesarum*, as if I was a caesar, not Charles.

The next couple of days were warm and fuzzy. We dined at the finest Roman restaurants and had dessert at my favorite café, Il Cigno. I started to worry if I'd gain twenty pounds in a week and not be prepared for the marathon. I googled a gym since I only run outside on race day. I was in luck. Just a five-minute drive, in the opposite direction of Rome, was another small town that had a gym. The plan was to go for a light three-mile run, then two miles the next day, then one mile the day before the marathon. I had no clue if this was a viable plan, but I felt it would help me stay warmed up for race day. Andrea asked if I wanted her to ride with me. I decided I'd go alone, not knowing how this decision could've changed the atmosphere of the week.

A concrete-reinforced steel gate opened to a neighborhood of villas. Caron's was at the top of a steep hill. Every day I drove the car out of the compound, I turned it around and drove out face first. But on this day, there were a lot of cars in the driveway. I decided it would be much easier to back out. Understand this, ladies and gentlemen of the jury: I don't drive a car every day, let alone a manual transmission. I only learned how to drive a manual when I lived in Italy ten years ago and only drove on visits to Europe, so I was rusty.

As I was rolling down the hill backward approaching a concrete wall at the end of the street, I didn't panic. I sat there processing how wonderful the trip had been so far. Gormandizing pasta dinners, floating past century-old churches to see old friends, the beauty of Rome, and the generosity of Caron. Everything had been going great up to this moment. "It's all downhill if I crash her car. How do you crash the car right in front of her house?" I whispered to myself.

It was an impossible situation. No hero was coming. I sat until I figured it out. I took a deep breath and channeled my inner Formula 1 racing champion Lewis Hamilton and started the engine. I clutched, I braked, I clutched and braked and gassed that puppy up—and in no time, I was on a treadmill at Evolution Fitness.

^^^

After three straight days running on the treadmill at *la palestra*, I was ready to hit the roads of *Roma*. I breezed through the expo looking for the bib pickup spot. But one vendor caught my eye. Two guys were standing behind a clamshell heat-press machine. The sign read *Metti il Tuo Nome a Maglietta*, which loosely translates to "Put your name on the shirt." My first thought was to correct his grammar, but my curiosity stopped me from insulting him. (*Metti il Tuo Nome Sulla Maglietta*, bro.) I was fascinated by the process and opportunity for a side hustle. I took him up on his offer, snapped a few pictures of his booth, and tucked that endeavor in my back pocket for later.

The race would be my first international marathon. As I rode in the Uber for the twenty minutes to the starting line, I pondered what one had to go through to run an international marathon. There's the flight, the hotel, the registration, miscellaneous transportation, and food: a $5,000 investment is a conservative number. Who gets to run around the globe? It is a heightened version of privilege. To understand the privilege, you only need to read anything beyond popular culture and sports. The assumption is that anyone can throw on a raggedy T-shirt and sneakers and run. But there are a few real barriers to running. If you take the time to consider what privilege means, you recognize that time to train is one major barrier. The cost of good running sneakers can be as high as $300. Additional accessories can also be in the hundreds. Race registration fees range from as little as $20 to as much as hundreds of dollars. But as noted, the costs for running the more prestigious races can be even higher than that.

The pouring rain didn't start immediately; rather, it waited to remind the runners who was really in control. I felt like a warrior right out the gate. The Colosseum to my left; the city of Rome to my right; in front of me, the path to victory; and behind me, the dust that some poor Italian would be eating. As I approached, I thought of the battles and the history of the Colosseum. Man versus man, man versus beast, and more—forms of entertainment that we would condemn today. My adidas Ultraboosts were struggling through their first marathon. The cobblestone, unevenly paved, ancient roads were as dichotomous as angels and demons—melting your heart as a tourist but scorching your soul as a marathoner. My feet began to throb only ten kilometers into the race.

The sky looked like a Dan Brown novel—dark, gloomy, and fictitious. Convective clouds dropped precipitation on my face at a rapid pace. I could barely see a few feet in front of me at times. My rain jacket was useless. I was soaked.

It's already been stated how much I love Italian culture. When I lived in Rome, I watched all the films, read all the newspapers, and was around a diverse group of Italians. It was only fitting that they'd be unique in how they organized their marathon. First, food is quite important to them. In order to appease the masses, they wouldn't dare offer artificial carbohydrate bars to supplement runners at aid stations; instead, there were tiny plates of pasta. I marveled over how infrequently you might see an Italian sweating, even in scorching heat. At every aid station were hundreds of thick yellow sponges—how dare they sweat during a forty-two-kilometer race. I guess that blew the budget—good luck finding a place to relieve yourself in the middle of the event. There were unwritten rules in place, like designated trees for men and women. And there were no facetious signs with witty lines to make you laugh, like: *If I see you collapse, I'll pause your Garmin; Remember, you paid for this* or; my favorite, *You're running better than our government.*

At around the eighteen-kilometer mark, the deep drumbeats of rain became light taps, more like brushstrokes on a high hat. Its timing couldn't have been more perfect. We were running up Via della Concilliazione, heading toward St. Peter's Square in Vatican City. I could see the Obelisco di Piazza San Pietro from a few blocks away. I turned off my music and took out my headphones.

"Che bello!," *"Grande San Pietro!,"* *"Che meraviglioso!,"* said the random runners. I needed to turn off Kanye and listen to my fellow marathoners, perhaps named Chiara and Gianpaolo, or any other random typical Italian name of today's local

marathoner. The Italian language is beautiful, and the people are warmhearted, generous, and proud. They were as excited to enter Vatican City as I was the first time I had seen it eight years ago. I stopped and got my portrait taken with runners and the square as my backdrop. At that moment, the pain in my feet ceased, and I reminisced about all the time I had spent in this square.

Soon we'd be arriving in my old neighborhood—Prati. I stopped again at the Lepanto subway station and snapped another picture. I had lived a block away during my first year in Italy. Toward the end of the race, we passed my other favorite squares: Piazza del Popolo and Piazza di Spagna. These were the two places I'd visit whenever I had nothing else to do on any particular day. I had also taken Italian lessons at a school near the Spanish Steps. Once we got to Piazza Venezia, that pretty much signaled the end of the race; we were at the forty-kilometer mark. The shower of rain splashed my face again. It rained so hard I felt like I was swimming. I rounded the corner to the finish. Now where were those sponges?

^^^

My performance wasn't bad, given the weather. I clocked my second-best time, just one minute behind the personal record I had set in Birmingham—and in a torrential downpour, no less. I made it back to Riano in one piece, showered, and changed clothes. Caron, Mauro, Andrea, and I went to the local jaunt that always rolled out the cherry-red carpet for Caron. I have a picture of me about to cut into a steak bigger than my torso. I guess they feed their cows pizza, pasta, and gelato instead of grass.

Two weeks after Rome, I would be running Boston. In the running community, the Boston Marathon was a mononym—like Oprah, Prince, or Madonna. All roads led to *Boston.*

Chapter 12
Patriots' Day, Boston.

After the resurgence of the marathon as the premier event at the modern Olympics, the city of Boston led the way for another movement, which spread the marathon to non-Olympic athletes. The Boston Marathon became an attraction for runners and non-runners alike, serving as a key stop for anyone who took the sport seriously. In 2013, however, something happened that would leave a mark on the history of the event.

The 117th Boston Marathon, run on Patriots' Day, April 15, was a raucous and joyous time, as Patriots' Day always is in Boston. Runner after runner crossed the finish line, the crowd cheering them on. At 2:49 p.m., however, those cheers turned into screams that would give pause to even the most exuberant runner's heart. A pair of blasts less than two hundred meters from the finish line silenced the spectators on Boylston Street.

It was pure horror and anguish. Here, people had joined from all around the world to watch and participate in the race of all races. Although the winner had already crossed the finish line, along with many other elite runners, thousands of others still lined the course from Beacon Street past Fenway Park and on to the finish line. For seven minutes, in the deadly confusion, the race clock continued to tick.

Three were dead, and another 265 from the crowd sustained injuries, fourteen of whom lost limbs. Many more, too many to count, would carry the psychological scars of that day with them for the rest of their lives. Everyone, from the first responders to the runners to the spectators to those who watched from afar on TV and internet streams, would remember the smoke billowing up Boylston Street.

Leaving behind their bags, the people in the crowd rushed to safety—at least, those who were able did. It was unclear which of those bags might contain another bomb. Fear filled the air on a day that was supposed to be one of the best of many people's lives, a day and a race for which they had trained and dreamed about.

One year later, at the 2014 Boston Marathon, the Eritrean American Keflezighi would cross the finish line with a time of 2:08:37. It would be the first time an American had won the Boston Marathon since 1983. On that Patriots' Day when the thirty-nine-year-old wore his gold medal, hearts and minds remembered those lost, the terror that all had felt when the brisk April air in Boston had turned to something more pernicious, and when it had seemed that the magic had been lost. Out of the tragedy, runners had reclaimed their most cherished race, ripping it from the hands of evil, holding always in their memory those lost that afternoon on Boylston Street.

I cried while watching the documentary, late 2016, detailing the horrific acts of that day. I cried even more afterward. I couldn't stop crying just thinking about it. Suddenly, a burning desire crept through the tears, and I knew only one thing: I had to run the Boston Marathon. I had no clue how challenging it was to obtain a place in the race. It was mid-November, just months before the 2017 Boston Marathon; certainly, all the spots were filled.

I must have made a hundred calls. Or at least it felt like it. Imagine Dave Chappelle giving his best setup; the punch line was my request for a race number. I was laughed at, hung up on, or silenced by a firm no about getting into the race. After calling most of the charity sponsors, I contacted Roxbury Community College. My tears crusted my face as I pleaded one final time while telling my story. "I just ran my second marathon. I'm home watching the marathon bombing documentary, and the pain I feel is driving me to participate in Boston."

There was a moment of silence until the man on the other end responded, "Go on . . ."

I thought, *Does this guy bask in pain? Is he going to laugh at me explaining my sadness?* I couldn't bear to be frustrated . . . I continued to almost beg for help.

We danced on the phone for an hour. I talked. He listened. He talked. I listened. And then we traded places like two pugilists exchanging blows. By the end of the call, I was the proud owner of the opportunity to raise $10,000 to support tuition at Roxbury Community College in exchange for a trip to the 2017 Boston Marathon. I say *opportunity* sarcastically, since I would have of course just wanted to pay the registration without begging friends and family for money yet again. It would be the 121st time in a row they would put on this competition. The longest continuous-running marathon in the world. In a few months, I would be running *Boston.*

^^^

Boston is the most coveted race for marathoners for many reasons. It was in 1897 that runners gathered on the starting line there for the first time. Only a year prior, the first Summer Olympics had featured a revival of the event in Athens. During all that time, the race evolved alongside marathoning, often influencing its development.

The first Boston Marathon was, for example, only 24.5 miles long. That was the length for twenty-seven years until organizers increased it to 26.2 miles in 1924 in accordance with the standard that the International Olympic Committee had set for the 1908 Summer Olympics. Pioneering the identity of marathon events as holidays and celebrations, the Boston Marathon would coincide every year with Patriots' Day. This holiday made sense on multiple fronts: the city was the traditional birthplace of the American Revolution, home of the Boston Massacre and the Boston Tea Party, congruent with the mythology behind the original marathon related to the Athenians' struggle for independence from the Persian Empire.

Every year since 1897, the Boston Marathon grew in popularity. What began as a New England tradition became a magnet for runners far and wide. Every marathoner wanted to run Boston. Within its first century, the event had become a must-run for professionals. It was because of their role in the race that the structure of the competition changed. Whereas locals and other amateurs had long accepted an olive branch wreath as the sole award, professional runners began to demand some sort of cash prize, which had become the norm at other major marathons.

The organizers of the Boston Marathon conceded to them. From 1986 onward, the winner would receive a monetary prize. It was around the same time that large corporations offered sponsorship deals for the race, both to the organizers and to the runners. The Boston Marathon became a place where the running community could come together—to see who the best was, to set expectations for the coming Olympics, and to synergize ideas and technologies emerging in the sport.

The culture around the Boston Marathon is distinctive. No other marathon, and few other sporting events, have managed to reach the level of phenomenon that it has. It is not only the first, but undoubtedly, it is the most important marathon. This race's history has helped shape its own sport—and left an imprint on all who have run it. This would no doubt be a formidable opponent.

Thanks to that good man at Roxbury Community College, as well as many of my friends and family (I raised the $10,000 for the school with their help), I secured a spot in the event. I was off to Beantown to the race expo. For five months, I had been working up the courage to tackle Heartbreak Hill. The wait was over. Because of the hills and stretches, most notably Heartbreak Hill on Commonwealth Avenue in Newton, many experienced runners have called the course among the most challenging in the world.

My adidas Ultraboosts were making their second appearance in a marathon, and my feet had barely recovered from the pounding they had taken running on the cobblestones in Italia. As for the rest of my body, it was running on pure adrenaline, and if pain existed, I didn't feel it.

I remember two major things on Andrea's and my trip to the race expo that Saturday afternoon before marathon Monday. The first was seeing so many runners with Boston jackets from years past. "So you've run Boston how many times?" I asked a guy who had sixteen different years embroidered onto a jacket from 1999.

He was tall, lanky, with brown, straight hair and blue eyes, around fiftyish. "Tomorrow will mark number seventeen, and I'll cross the finish line even if it kills me," he muttered with an air of certitude.

I saw jackets from last year, from the nineties, from the eighties, and more.

"I guess the jacket is a big thing," I said to one runner.

"It's more important than the medal. It's a badge of honor that you can wear forever any day of the week," replied the thirtyish female with a shot-putter-esque body.

I was certainly going to get a jacket, but not until I got the medal. I'm just a little superstitious.

The other thing that caught my attention was the classified section in the back with a sign that read ABBOTT WORLD MARATHON MAJORS. It felt so exclusive and elusive. I walked over to the booth and started talking to the rep. "What is this marathon majors all about?" I asked.

She seemed so tired of that question that she merely pointed to the informative sign next to her. It was like I was in an art gallery in Chelsea, and the *gallerina*, who plays a mute, never utters a word when you're lucky enough to have been allowed inside. Apparently, the Abbott World Marathon Majors is a series of the largest, most renowned marathons in the world: Berlin, Boston, Chicago, London, New York City, and Tokyo.

"Oh great. Something else for you to sink your teeth into," Andrea said with a slight bit of sarcasm mixed with enthusiasm.

I had no clue whether I was interested in anything other than walking around with my unicorn medal from my neck for a day. Focus . . . Boston.

The grandeur and parade of the Boston Marathon is something to behold. The start is far outside the city. We boarded a shuttle and bused out to the start in Hopkinton, Massachusetts. When we arrived, a runner named Belma Mendez, a native Bostonian of Ecuadorian descent, approached me. How she spotted me in the swarming crowd of people, I have no idea. But our bib numbers were only one number apart, so she had a suspicion that I was also sponsored by her employer, Roxbury Community College.

"Do you work for RCC?" she asked with a smile so big you couldn't help but be warmed by it.

"No, I raised money for the school and received this opportunity in exchange," I responded.

She had been a fan of the race as a spectator for years. "I watched the Boston Marathon ten years in a row and left the bombing area because my daughter was tired," she said. "It was only minutes before the first bomb went off."

I started to wonder what could've been for Belma and her daughter. We high-fived and decided we were going to start the race together. She had immigrated from Ecuador in 1993. Running Boston was a dream come true after watching it for so many years and later recovering from the trauma she had felt after so many innocent spectators and runners had their lives changed in 2013.

Around three miles in, we were passing Ashland. Belma was fast. I noticed she was slowing her pace to let me keep up. I gracefully acknowledged this and told her she should run her race and we could exchange numbers and catch up at the finish line. So, at around the 10K mark in Framingham, we gave one last high-five, and she pressed the turbo button and was off.

Your gear is so important. By the time I got to Lake Cochituate, around mile nine, I already was hitting a wall. My feet felt like I had been walking through the Gobi Desert at midday ... barefoot. I had taped my legs, hips, and ankles with KT Tape, but I may as well have used BAND-AIDs. Not to mention that I was tasting the salt in my sweat, and I had forgotten my salt sticks to balance my electrolytes. It was way too early to be crashing, and in two minutes flat I was certainly popping an Advil, which I normally took around mile twenty-two. But I looked like a million bucks. Boston colors are yellow and blue with black trim. I wore a peacock-blue lululemon top, ebony-black lululemon tights, and my adidas Ultraboosts were sapphire blue with a canary-yellow side patch. Oh, and a GoPro chest harness was strapped on me. I was going to look good if I had to catch my first DNF.

I began to hear shrill wailing—kvlt screams, pigs squealing, babies yelling, well-enunciated lyrics. But there was no heavy-metal band, farm animals, or daycares. I was entering the scream tunnel in Wellesley. As legendary as Wellesley's alumni are the ladies who roar while lining the wall five deep like a packed stadium. Hundreds of students gather every year to cheer on the runners, and I think we were all looking forward to it on that hot April day. The students hand make the signs, many at the requests of runners. It's a tradition that has gone on for decades and is even listed on Wellesley's website as one of the things you must do before graduating. It's emotionally energizing. Perfect timing for runners like me hitting a wall about five miles too early.

I remembered all the things I had heard about Heartbreak Hill. "People tap out at Heartbreak Hill," my friend Matt told me about a week before the race. In one online article, a run coach exclaimed, "You need to train for Heartbreak Hill!" Heartbreak Hill? Well, I've got news for you. I remembered the Death March, just seven months ago, making grown men and women cry. What's a hill to a mountain? If Heartbreak Hill brought you to tears, the Death March was a full-on catastrophic meltdown.

I felt so good at that moment that I didn't even notice my music was off. I flipped the switch and went into beautiful, dark, twisted fantasy mode.

The roads during Boston looked to me like I owned them. I made my way up Beacon Street, passing Commonwealth Avenue, and stopped the moment I arrived at the final stretch: Boylston Street.

I slowed my pace to a gliding walk. I looked myself up and down. I admired my choice of gear. I looked like a star. As a child, I had wanted to compete in the most prestigious academic tournaments at the city, state, and national levels. I had found it challenging to learn Italian while studying in Perugia and Rome. As an adult, I had wanted to attend Harvard University for the prestige of the degree. Now, marathoning placed goals like Boston in front of me. It had been the backdrop of my most admired university—between the two was the Charles River—and conquering it was Charles.

I later learned that my new friend Belma crossed the finish line after me. She had broken down eight hundred meters from the finish and had to be carried across. There were images of her with her medal, all smiles, but in a wheelchair. She made a full recovery. But my time was better than hers.

^^^

Within moments of completing the race, I was all smiles on the phone with my mom. "Wow, you just ran Boston," she said. A year ago, she wouldn't have known what that had even meant. But there were those who were watching me on this journey. Some admired my will, others were inspired by my victories; my mom was proud of my courage.

Andrea's longtime friend Carol joined us at the MET Back Bay on Dartmouth Street to celebrate. Carol—a retail executive, Massachusetts native, and all-around fan of anything sports- and Boston-related—was so excited for me. "First glass of champagne is on me!" she joyfully announced upon arrival. Then Carol whispered, "Okay, what was your time?"

"I don't know exactly, but I'm sure I came in first," I joked.

Always the serious one about her Boston sports, she didn't laugh. Carol looked at Andrea with an approving smile. "You must be proud of this guy right now. He just finished Boston."

We all sat in silence for a few moments, then continued to drink our champagne.

Chapter 13

Bridges!

The Andy Warhol Museum has always been on my to-do list, but the six-hour drive from New York City had always dissuaded me ... That is, until now: I was going to run the Pittsburgh Marathon. The trouble was, I was tired before I even got there. We were into the fifth month of the year, and I had already run five marathons. This would be my sixth. Andrea was returning to glory, running the half-marathon. And we were going to the City of Bridges in Western Pennsylvania.

The last few months had been spent researching clamshell presses, precut vinyl letters and numbers, and how deeply we wanted to get into starting a race vendor side business. I chose a brand called Stahls' because it is pretty much the Mercedes-Benz of manual heat-transfer press machines. I called it "the changemaker." If I had only looked past that booth in Rome on marathon day, we wouldn't be about to make all this money. "How about we just quit our jobs now?" I said with a laugh.

Andrea, always the sensible one, replied, "We'll wait until after our first million, then we'll quit. That shouldn't take us longer than a few weeks."

I was surprised at how serious she sounded. In no time, I was down $12,000 on this investment and on the road early to the Pittsburgh Marathon party. We arrived in a city that reminded me of Amsterdam: lots of bridges, tall people, and bikes. We decided to take a drive through the city and let Google be our unpaid guide.

The Allegheny River is not exactly a river in the true sense of the word. It is a stream, all 325 miles of it, officially deemed an offshoot of the Ohio River. The Allegheny has shaped the Steel City into one of countless bridges that are emblematic of the type of acceptance and grace that are core to Pittsburgh's character.

The Liberty Bridge, at 2,663 feet high, is one of the larger bridges, but shorter than the 3,750-foot Homestead Grays Bridge. The Roberto Clemente Bridge, named for the Hall of Fame baseball player and Pittsburgh Pirates standout, has become something of a tourist spot. Similar in height is the Andy Warhol Bridge, named for another of the city's most cherished native sons. There is the Rachel Carson Bridge, commemorating the marine biologist's pioneering conservation work.

I pondered why renowned African American playwright August Wilson was missing from that list. I thought of the god of beginnings, endings, and passages—like bridges. How could Janus forget the writer of the collective about this town, *The Pittsburgh Cycle*? I thought about all the African Americans forgotten here. I thought about the high rate of coronary disease in areas like Allegheny County, the predominantly Black community, with the highest levels of air pollution. What would

Wilson's eleventh play have been about? Maybe the unequal treatment in Pittsburgh's housing, education, and economic systems? Maybe he would have written about a father teaching his son about the importance of running and how it strengthens your cardiovascular system? We cross every bridge as we come to it. On that Thursday before the race, I would be crossing both the bridge to become a race expo entrepreneur and all the bridges that make up part of the marathon course.

At the Pittsburgh Marathon expo, located downtown, we strolled up to the vendor entrance, visibly beating our chests as if all the money coming through this site was ours. "The New Yorkers have arrived," I joked with the security guard.

After setting up, Andrea and I stared at each other in silence with a fear that was hard to describe. It was like we had just been told to climb Mount Everest with nothing more than the clothes on our backs and the equipment at this booth. "What the heck are we doing?" I mumbled to myself.

The doors opened. Hundreds of the five thousand expected racers poured into the expo. We had the perfect location. Everyone running had to pass us to get their T-shirts and race bibs. One by one, they stopped by with generous smiles—and then passed us by.

We started naming our targets between us. "What, Jessica? Don't you want people to know who you are?" Andrea said with a smirk.

"Come on, Billy, you can do it. Step up to the plate and come pay me thousands. I got five on it," I whispered.

We needed to sweeten the deal. I thought about running to Whole Foods and getting a bottle of honey to spread all over our booth.

On day one, Friday, we made $600 in sales—well on our way to that first million. Day two, Saturday, was much more eventful. Friday was like a test run, a sprint, because the short window to sell in the expo was so small, given that the local runners could only come after work. On Saturday, it was more like a marathon— we had all day to work our business magic. Swarms of runners made their way in the door. Our faces were wide with smiles; we had our cake and were ready to eat it too. But the knell seemed more fitting for a funeral than the announcement that we'd be breaking Ken Jennings's record on *Jeopardy!* I almost didn't even want to tally the winnings.

"What's the take?" Andrea asked.

I counted. I recounted. "We were robbed. We're short about $996,850."

When it comes to my time as a race expo "Name on your T-shirt" vendor, I'm the winner of the Henri de Toulouse-Lautrec award. Jesus wept.

Meanwhile, I switched my shoes back to HOKA Bondis because they're also good for walking. The internal bruising at the bottom of my feet had begun to heal, my joints felt great, and my morale was high. I looked at my checklist and went shopping at the expo. I had to replenish my supplies of KT Tape, Honey Stinger Energy Chews, salt sticks, Nuun electrolyte tablets, and Advil after pretty much every major race. I also had to give myself a pep talk because in the back of my head was always the concern that this could be the day. The day I received my first DNF. *I know the Lord ain't brought me this far just to drop me off here . . . Did I make myself clear?* My doubts were always concealed by my unwavering confidence. Andrea said I was born to do incredible feats. Sure, she was midway through a nap when she said it, but I repeated, *I was born to do incredible feats.*

The evening before the race, we found an Italian restaurant with the highest rating in the city. "You'd have to cross hundreds of bridges to get better pizza and pasta," one of the reviews read. We were sold. We piled into our rental car and headed over to load up on carbohydrates. We were looking for an edge. The place was filled with runners. I could tell because half the diners were toting clear plastic bags filled with a T-shirt, race bib, and a timing chip. I can't lie; I was looking for familiar faces. Faces of marathoners who would be running with our vinyl on their backs. I saw none. I kept it simple and ordered a Margherita pizza. Andrea, on the other hand, got fancy and wanted some protein; she ordered the white pizza with clams and pancetta. Sometimes the only way to find the edge is to go over it.

^^^

We woke up Sunday at 5 a.m., got dressed, and were out the door without a hitch. *We* were running together for the first time in a major race; I was running the full marathon, and Andrea was running the half. The race was like another world. I could sense a bit of nervousness from Andrea. She's usually pretty cool, but she was complaining about aches before we started. "I feel like my knee might not hold up," she blurted out.

I felt like she would be okay. Especially since she is a much more disciplined person than I, which carries over to her training style. "You'll be fine. You've trained for this, and it's not your first rodeo," I reassured her.

The racecourse was impressive, complex, and challenging. Lots of direction changes, running over bridges, and ungodly puffs of smoke from industrial facilities. I didn't know much about the city of Pittsburgh, aside from it contributing to a memorable scene in the film *Goodfellas*. Henry Hill, the film's protagonist, talks about his Pittsburgh connection. Pittsburgh is also known for the Wiz Khalifa song "Black and Yellow" and, of course, all its championship-winning sports teams.

Andrea and I ran the first ten miles together, which was calming to just casually chat while keeping a steady pace. Although I had run a few marathons at this point, I was never a consistent trainer. This showed next to someone who pretty much based her running style on consistency. It wasn't her speed that I was having a hard time keeping up with, but rather her consistent, nonstop, placid tempo. "You have such a smooth stride," I said. I figured if I overcomplimented her, it might distract her from seeing that I was struggling to glide across the 412.

By mile eight, reality started to sink in. What had initially felt like an easy run in the park became an actual marathon. I broke stride and started to walk. "Go on ahead of me. Don't worry, I'll catch up," I said, gasping for air.

The New York City Marathon was the only race during which I had felt joyous the entire time. That's not to say it wasn't difficult or challenging, but rather that I had been so eager to cross that finish line for the first time, I had skipped, I had danced, I had even done push-ups in the middle of that race. But every marathon afterward, there was some point where I asked myself, "Why are you here again?" And I responded to myself every time, "We're never doing this again." I wanted to say it aloud to Andrea. I wouldn't find out till later how much she was struggling. And she definitely had no clue how much I was struggling. We were like two bees, failing at secreting enough beeswax to make a honeycomb: bordering on uselessness. We started to walk. We both popped an Advil, hoping it would subdue the mental pain of us failing at our business venture and then bombing the race.

We walked for ten minutes, but it felt like an eternity. Luckily, the Advil felt like it was kicking in. "How are you feeling?" Andrea shouted, not realizing I had turned off my music.

I stretched my shoulders and started to think about what the finisher's medal would look like. I thrust my legs in the air, performing high knees as if I were warming up. I raised both arms in the air, remembering Sylvester Stallone's iconic pose when he reached the top of the Philadelphia Museum of Art steps in the first *Rocky* film. Then I thought about a real American hero, Todd Beamer, and turned to Andrea. "Let's roll."

All pain was gone. All doubts became certainty. We slapped a high-five and got back in the race. We had two miles to go before we'd part. The half-marathoners turned left on their final three miles, and the marathoners kept straight for another sixteen. We hugged and were off to finish our respective courses.

^^^

During the rest of the race, I put on some music, and it felt like I was sailing off the coast of Porto Cervo on the island of Sardinia in Italy: effortless. I crossed the finish line expecting to see Andrea but didn't spot her. I made my usual first call to my mother and told her about the race while walking the quarter of a mile toward the hotel. Simultaneously, I was sending text messages to Andrea with no response. It was then that I felt a rush of blood to my head, and I sensed something was awry. I walked into the hotel room to find her fast asleep. I let out a chuckle and started making noises to wake her up.

"Don't turn on the lights," she groaned. I realized she had closed the blinds, the lights were off, and her entire body was submerged beneath a sea of blankets. Upon entering the bathroom, I smelled traces of last night's pizza, which must have decided it was not happy with a half-marathon run.

My next thought was to rummage through the room for a half-marathon medal that one would receive when they *finished* the race. The pounding in my chest, indicating I was worried about my wife's spirit if she had received a DNF, was placated once I saw a large, round medal draped over her vendor lanyard that read *DICK's Sporting Goods Pittsburgh Half Marathon 2017 Finisher*. My next thought was, *I guess I'll be driving us home.* We skipped the Andy Warhol Museum and decided to just head home.

Summer break begins early for me. Most marathons are in the beginning and end of the year, and I hate running in the heat. I had four months until the next marathon. The fall would be nothing less than the equivalent of a Mount Everest climbing season. I was going to run five marathons, every two weeks, from September 24 to November 19.

Chapter 14

Berlin & Rosa...

B erlin was a trip—in more ways than one. It would be my second international marathon and third Abbott World Marathon Majors event. I was beginning to think that running all six majors was feasible. This was also the fourth major race for which I had to raise money in order to gain a spot. I trolled social media, texted and called friends, and even threw a fundraising party.

I only needed eight hundred bucks for this, a far cry from the $10,000 I had needed for Boston and the four grand I had needed for New York City. But still, I figured I'd try to have a little fun. I invited a few friends over with the hope that they would donate to the fundraiser, and I'd soon be off to devour schnitzel and sauerkraut, and wash it all down with a hefeweizen.

As it goes, I have a few friends who love to travel. Shircara, a thirtysomething senior project manager at Pfizer, had already booked a trip to Berlin. She held a seat on the New York Cares Junior Board alongside Andrea, and we developed a friendship after she became one of my clients. While on a call discussing her account, we realized we'd be passing like ships in the night, as she would be arriving just days after I would be departing. If I ran as fast as she changed her plans, I'd probably be walking up to the pole, placing within the top three. We had only realized the day before taking off that we would be on the same flight.

Alessandro, who is based in Rome, always loved visiting Germany. He and I had been talking about him running a marathon with me ever since my photo finish in Italia a few months ago. You could throw a rock from Rome and hit Berlin; it felt so close. Nonstop flights ran frequently, and you could touch down in two hours flat. Alessandro didn't think twice about meeting me and decided that he'd share a room with Shircara, although they had never met.

Jayson, a banker at JP Morgan, was a friend whom I had met in grad school back in 2008. On the first day of class, he walked up to me and said, "You're the only other Black guy I've seen, so I guess I'd better introduce myself." He spent a semester in Rome on my suggestion and couldn't stop thinking about Europe after that. He knew Alessandro well. When I returned to New York City, Jayson and I were inseparable for at least the first year. On one occasion, we were at a networking event and he popped out for a smoke break, where he met a real estate broker and native New Yorker named Marie. They ended up becoming BFF's, and Marie became part of my tribe as well. Jayson and Marie were attending a wedding in Milan and would make their way to Berlin right afterward.

On our Delta flight from New York City to Berlin, we sat in the rear of coach, drooling over the entrées Shircara was getting in first class. "I only fly business," she would remind us upon landing.

We had a brief layover in Amsterdam. I have no clue why I started video recording. "What's your name?" I announced with the camera pointed to Shircara.

"My name is Shircara, and I'm a Black girl rocking in Amsterdam. And argh, it's six a.m.!"

"My name is Andrea; are we there yet?" Andrea said. She loves traveling but hates the travel part.

It wouldn't be long before we would be doing this dance again at the airport in Berlin. As we approached baggage claim, I was stopped by a passenger not from our plane. He was a thirtysomething, thin, Black male with thick glasses and looked a lot like an Ivy League physics professor. "E-e-excuse m-m-me. I n-n-noticed your Boston j-j-jacket and wanted to know if y-y-you knew where we go to get our r-r-race materials?" he asked with a nervous stutter.

Could it be? Another Black man running an international marathon? I thought. I whipped out my phone and helped him with the directions. "Where are you from?" I asked.

"London," he said with a thick British accent. I had first thought he might be Caribbean and living in America, but he was closer to his own neck of the woods.

DJ, my younger brother, had arrived two days before us to scope the place out. He picked us up from the airport in a Mercedes SUV. Shircara, Andrea, DJ, and I made our way back to the Moxy Berlin Ostbahnof Hotel, where we would wait for Alessandro, Marie, and Jayson to arrive. After waiting hours for a response, we realized Jayson and Marie were clearly not going to show up in time to visit the expo with us. We piled into DJ's Benz and made our way downtown. We were all ravenous after traveling and decided we would get my race number and grab

something quick to eat at the expo. As we were walking through
to take pictures, I stumbled across the Black gentleman from the
airport. "You found your way over here!"

"Why is a Black dude from London running the Berlin
Marathon?" I asked.

Andrew, who has shaved off about one hundred pounds since
2012 while running in eleven marathons and receiving numerous
medals for other races. In the coming weeks I would learn more
about Andrew's background. He shared his compelling story
with me in an email:

Ever since I was a kid in elementary school, I enjoyed
competing against my peers in running events. I relished the
longer and muddier challenge of a 5km cross country event,
however, my teachers regularly reminded me that my Jamaican
heritage allegedly made me more suitable for the 100m sprint
event. I remember doing a Robin Hood charity event in my
hometown of Nottingham while I was still at elementary school.
I'm guessing it was about 10km or more, but long enough for
me to puke my guts out as I crossed the finish line and that was
enough to make me think long distance runners were all nuts
and that put me off forever. That is until my late mother got
diagnosed with cancer.

The Marie Curie nurses that helped our family look after
mum were amazing, but she didn't make it and her loss shook
me and I entered a state of depression. It was at this point in my
life in March 2013, as an overweight, 37-year-old, married father
of three children that I turned back to running. I trained and ran
half-marathons to raise money for Marie Curie nurses, a charity
my late mum also did voluntary work for before she became ill.

Some of those running events were in very rural areas of England, where not only was I viewed with suspicion for being the only Black guy at the event, but often spectators would stop applauding as I ran past and then [return] to applaud[ing] white runners behind me. At first, I thought I was imagining this occurrence until I came across other Black runners recalling the same experience. Rather than put me off, such pathetic discrimination put fire in my belly, and I now had my ambition set on doing a full marathon, as I could also see the benefit running was having on my physical and mental health. I completed my first marathon aged 40. In the same year I did the Athens Marathon 2016 (OG!); by then I had the running bug, and I had my sights set not just on completing more marathons to raise money for charities, but also on achieving the coveted Abbott's World Marathon Majors Six Star medal.

To earn the Six Star Medal a marathoner must run a total of 157.2 miles across 6 cities, 4 countries and 3 continents! The medal is so exclusive that more people have climbed to the top of Mount Everest...

I looked for Black role models in the UK that had achieved it and found none; however, I'd been here before: I've been the first Black guy or family member known to me to do this or that and it didn't faze me then and wasn't going to faze me now.

The earliest major marathon of the six, Berlin, also happened to be the 2nd closest to me, so I trained hard and jetted off for the Berlin Marathon 2017. Berlin is where ... I instinctively gravitated toward [Charles] and his team to swap contact details and to learn about his "why." Berlin is also where I first laid my eyes on a real version of the Abbott's 6 Star medal and I have never looked back since...

When potential Black runners look at the field of participants and they see me as "one of only a few" or "the only" or "the first" in the context of Black people at an event, they will hopefully no longer see that as a barrier for them, but as an opportunity.

^^^

At the BMW Berlin Marathon was where I experienced several firsts. In the parking lot of my hotel, I met my first wheelchair racer. Hans, a Munich resident also staying at the Moxy, was about to finish his tenth marathon. After being diagnosed with multiple sclerosis, he took to participating in the distance race to find the meaning behind his prognosis. "I try to remain positive, and racing gives me a rush that can't be replicated," he told me and Alessandro. His words inspired me.

On race day, I met up with Jenine. Her cousin had introduced us a few months ago, knowing that we would both be two random Black people ceaselessly galloping through Berlin and that we should probably meet, if not for anything else but to give each other the nod on our way past the starting line. After making the fifty-three-hundred-mile trip, Jenine arrived in Berlin with a unique story:

I ran my first marathon in 2007, my youngest son was 2 years old, and I still had not lost the "baby weight" I gained while pregnant with him. I was motivated to try running to drop the extra pounds.

I'd known people who had run races (working in the corporate world) marathon racing, really any endurance sport, made for great cubicle conversations. I was inspired by people's stories but never thought I could or would finish a race myself.

My older cousin, Andrea, who introduced me to Charles, had run the New York Marathon and her experiences and stories, plus the great shape she was in, inspired me to register for my first race. Crossing that first finish line at the Houston Marathon was a proud moment, and truthfully it was also a disaster . . . I learned all the hard lessons about finding better training & nutrition plans, breaking in race gear ahead of time, blister protection, all the things! I was much better prepared for the four marathons and many half-marathons, 10k and 5k races that I've run since then.

In researching races after that first one, I discovered the world majors and that became a bucket list item for me to complete over the course of my lifetime!

Aside from staying fit and maintaining a consistent workout routine, running and finishing races has given me the confidence and mental toughness to achieve in all areas of life. Personally and professionally. So many of the characteristics and attributes that it takes to be successful in running carry over and really become a metaphor for life . . .

And race spectators with their cheers and sign slogans always put a smile on my face, even on the dreaded mile 22 of a race. There is an instant and lasting connection among runners . . . Though the sport is more mainstream and diverse than it was 16 years ago . . . there is more that can be done to expose African American men and women to endurance racing as a form of regular exercise. I often am the only minority at most race start lines . . .

Perhaps the sharing of success stories, and a living example of people enhancing quality of life through running is a step in the right direction.

Next to Jenine and I stood Jessica, a thirtysomething blonde and blue-eyed American sporting a green poncho and a smile bigger than the Berlin TV Tower. I noticed a bulge in her stomach and couldn't resist a question.

"What's that thing under your poncho?" Jenine asked, beating me to the punch.

"It's my baby," she responded as if she couldn't wait to show it off. She lifted her poncho, and her black T-shirt read *Baby's First Marathon: Berlin 2017*. A heart underneath it had one-half of the American flag, and the other half was the German flag.

I couldn't believe it. I was so inspired. I had met my first racer who was bound to a wheelchair, and now I had met a woman seven months pregnant. Jessica and I snapped a selfie, and we were off to the races soon enough.

I had made another footwear change on this race and went from the heavier HOKA Bondis to the sleeker, lighter Cliftons. I'd like to say my choice came from calculated research, but really, the chunky heels just made me feel old. And the Cliftons seemed made for a gentleman who is still able to have dinner after five, doesn't use a landline phone, and hasn't had his license taken away from him due to him totally not seeing STOP signs. My race plan was simple. I'd trained. I'd run eight marathons, two of them Abbott World Marathon Majors, and all I needed to do was cross the finish line. I've always known there could be up to a million spectators at any race, but now I felt under a microscope with a team that had traveled thousands of miles to see me run. And to party afterward.

I started slow and steady. I ran a thirty-four-minute 5K, which was minutes slower than my typical run, but I didn't want to come out too hot. Runners that sprint out of the gate risk hitting their proverbial wall early. As the old saying goes, it's a marathon, not a sprint. With all things that take time in life, you have to pace yourself and be patient. By the time I reached the half-marathon point, I was tracking a five-hour marathon. The Berlin crew, most of whom had been out until 6 a.m. enjoying the cultural artifacts of the city (i.e., drinking copious amounts of beer), decided they would finally join Andrea and Marie by mile fourteen. DJ, always looking for an angle, knew exactly how to maneuver the winding roads (under Andrea's expert directing skills, of course) to find me.

They would see me a total of four times during that race, and I must say it made me proud. Here I was, this kid from Detroit, with an entire entourage cheering me on as I trucked along a forty-two-kilometer run. At the finish line, I couldn't help remembering Ronald Reagan's 1987 speech that called for the fall of the Berlin Wall. I was now passing the very spot: the Brandenburg Gate. That evening, we partied like rock stars as the DJ spun German punk mixed with American hip-hop.

^^^

Culturally, Berlin had a lot to offer. A few months earlier, I'd read an article about Ryan Mendoza, an American artist who had relocated his studio there. As a visionary, he often took on large-scale projects that no one wanted to fund. One of them was the restoration and maintenance of the Rosa Parks home.

Parks was a civil rights pioneer who entered the public sphere when she refused to vacate her bus seat in deference to a White passenger. Born to a Black family in rural Alabama, she grew up near Ku Klux Klan territory and consistently experienced the threat of violence and oppression. In 1955, Parks—then a Montgomery resident—rose to acclaim when she disobeyed the bus driver's orders to move to the back of a segregated bus. Parks was ultimately arrested, yet she became a near-instant icon as a result of her measured defiance, spearheading the Montgomery bus boycott as a result. This incident marked one of many acts of resistance; Parks had repeatedly ignored bus segregation rules over the course of many years, voicing her beliefs in the form of nonviolent protest.

Parks and her family relocated to Detroit in 1957. She stayed involved with the NAACP for most of her life. She received the Congressional Gold Medal of Honor in 1999—the highest honor a civilian can be awarded in the United States—setting an example for her contemporaries and future generations. Upon her passing in 2005, my mother and brother attended her funeral. "To this day, the picture of Mom and me after the Parks funeral is my favorite of us," DJ would later confide in me. He and I were now about to become the first visitors from Detroit, the artist would tell us, to see her home reconstructed by Mendoza in Germany's capital city. The home was about to be demolished when Ryan Mendoza purchased it, deconstructed it, and moved it to his property, at the permission of Parks' family. It was an emotional feeling for me.

The home itself looked like a Roy Lichtenstein sculpture. The black-and-white color scheme seemed timeless, as if it predated color photography from the late 1890s. The half-painted wood shingles left us wondering whether this was the original paint job—a question typical of DJ, who loves the nostalgia of classic vehicles, and me, who loves the patina of vintage timepieces. My favorite picture of this trip is of us in front of house number 267.

Parks's defiance and courage was felt around the world. Her legacy remains embodied not only by what she chose not to do, but also by how her acts presented a new way of understanding the multiplicity and diversity of Blackness. If I only had half the strength and tenacity as she, I'd inspire a few more men and women. I was about to go to Chicago with a backpack full of emotions.

Chapter 15

The Lioness Roars.

Growing up in Detroit, I always had ties to Chicago. It was less than three hundred miles away and was an easy road trip for us. My mother loved eating at the Navy Pier restaurants, shopping on the Magnificent Mile, and admiring the beauty of the city's architecture. Although the Detroit Pistons were the team of the mid- to late eighties in the NBA, I was a die-hard Jordan fan, and that led me to support the red and black. And frankly speaking, it was my kind of town.

Ever since the Great Migration, Chicago has served as one of the cradles of Black culture and heritage in America. Here, music has flourished, and in recent decades, new art forms, including improv and stand-up comedy, have emerged. However, the city has taken on another, less favorable significance as well: it is the epicenter of some of the most disheartening and horrific realities of life for Black Americans.

Before we can delve into these issues, we need to consider some of the local history. Throughout the 1910s, while Black families moved out of the South and into the Midwest, lynching became more common. In 1919, after a group of White swimmers murdered a Black child by assaulting him with rocks because he had (accidentally or not) broken the segregation line, the Chicago Riot broke out. Black protesters filled the beaches of Lake Michigan, and White mobs lashing out at the protestors committed more violence. When the rioting ended after two weeks, twenty-three Black people had died. Black Chicagoans went homeless on a huge scale: more than one thousand Black families were out on the streets in the weeks that followed.

Today, we are witnessing up close the inevitable results of atrocities like this one and of the broken system that those atrocities represented. According to one study published by NPR, Black people living in majority-Black neighborhoods can expect a lifespan thirty years shorter than their White counterparts living in majority-White neighborhoods. This is more shocking when one realizes that the Chicago counties in question—Streeterville and Englewood—are barely ten miles away from each other.

Race is the determining factor in this situation: 103 years ago in Chicago, you were more likely to die or go homeless due to the riots if you were Black, just as today in the city, if you are Black, you can assume you are not going to live as long. On average, in this neighborhood, you won't even live long enough to collect Social Security.

Those who have left the city have tried to make sense of what happened. At one time, Chicago would have seemed like the promised land to Black former sharecroppers and slaves escaping the bonds of Mississippi, Alabama, Louisiana, and Georgia. Linda Villarosa, a journalist whose family moved her from Chicago to a Colorado suburb when she was ten years old, says of the problem, "These neighborhoods lack resources. They lack grocery stores. They lack healthy outdoor space. They often lack clean air and clean water and clean land. If you live in a place like that—that has few resources but also worse conditions—your health suffers."

As these health issues become more apparent and they begin to claim more lives, it is important to ask what response would be both appropriate and effective. Any such conversation will necessarily turn to reparations. Just as tobacco companies have paid settlements for the harm they have caused their customers by knowingly and intentionally selling harmful products, there is a list of organizations, beginning with the state and federal governments, that should work to rectify this injustice.

Chicago may never hold the shine that it once did for a downtrodden people seeking respite in a place far different from the pains they had left behind. However, it can still become a place of hope. It can take on a new significance as a healer and as a leader, as a force to ensure that what is right will be done and the past is never painted over. I hope the Chicago Marathon race directors are listening.

I called my mother after every marathon I ran—even when I was crossing the finish line in a time zone that had me six hours away. This time, I was calling her to come and see me run in person for the first time. "This race is on October 8," I said. Giving her no time for a rebuttal, I sweetened the prospect, assuring her I'd be covering her stay at the W Hotel with points.

"Maybe," she said, and I could sense her smiling through the phone. I also suggested she bring my nephew, Jaron—Hazel's youngest son. He was coming to the age where I felt I could inspire that next generation of Moore men to burst through the tape and be presented with a marathon medal.

My mother and I have always had a special bond. She was quite young when I was born, and I'm the oldest of her four children. She has always been my number one fan and supporter for everything I've done, no matter how eccentric and weird. As she'd put it, "That's just Charles." I always viewed her as an ambitious Black woman, assertive and loyal: a typical Scorpio. When I was a kid, her eyes would light up as she talked about the real estate properties she owned and all the others she planned to buy. I became a second-generation art collector on the shoulders of my mom. She never intended to be a collector. She just wanted to decorate her home with Black artists who painted the Black experience. Her pride and satisfaction with her acquisitions always stuck with me.

Andrea and I arrived in Chicago the Friday before the marathon after a two-hour flight. As soon as I got to the hotel room, I put my camera phone on video selfie mode and started singing, "My kind of town, Chicago is . . ." My mom and Jaron arrived later that afternoon via car.

After lunch, Andrea and I rushed over to the expo, late of course, and snatched my race packet. I knew that Cathy, my friend from New York City whom I'd met in Orlando, would be there. *Where are you?* I typed into my phone. She called me right back, and I saw her waving at me from across the convention center. When you're in a different city among a sea of runners, it's always great to see a familiar face. And although your friends and family are important supporters, it's no substitute for those who are physically in the trenches with you. Cathy is a fiftyish-year-old native New Yorker who works as an accountant for a real estate developer. We had run a couple of 5Ks together; we clocked a similar pace and traveled a lot for races. I always loved her energetic, positive spirit when it comes to life and marathoning.

Chicago was insanely hot for October. By noon, it had gotten up to eighty-one degrees. Ideal marathon weather for me hovers around fifty degrees. A 2014 *Runner's World* article, "What's the Optimal Temperature for Marathons?," discussed this very subject. According to a group of French researchers who analyzed 1.8 million finishing time results in a ten-year block, 43.2 degrees was the magic number. Upon further analysis, the best times were when the weather didn't top forty degrees. It makes sense that even when joking around at Disney, I ran one of my better times when we had sub-forty-degree temperatures.

I glanced over at Cathy's face at the start, and she didn't look happy. "How is it this hot in the Windy City this time of year?" she blurted out.

Back at my first race in New York City, the temperature had peaked around fifty-five and had dropped down to the low forties for most of that race. "Why can't Chicago be more like New York?" I griped.

Chicago is always *trying* to be like New York City when it comes to marathoning. In the 1970s, the sport was not very popular among amateurs, and Manhattan would hold the entire race in Central Park. In the eighties, New York City Marathon cofounder Fred Lebow and Chicago Marathon race director Bob Bright publicly traded jabs on which race was the premier event. Bright hilariously said to a reporter that he'd make Lebow switch to a spring race in order to not have to compete with Chicago for elite participants. Since it was too late to take the title of longest continuous race—Boston being far ahead—the cities began to volley for the status as the largest in the world.

As of today, New York City reigns as the largest race field in the world, but Chicago is one of the Abbott World Marathon Majors. But as we were gearing up to start, it was clear to Cathy and me which was the leader in our book. "I'll take sixty or even seventy degrees," I complained.

I was far enough from the frontrunners that the gun blast signaling the race start sounded muffled. We took off. "Don't come out too hot," Cathy warned.

She had been running for years and had much more experience than I, but I knew exactly what she meant. I slowed my pace to match hers. But around mile two, she was already crashing. The heat was not friendly to her. I ignored the brutal sun shamelessly pummeling me with its rays. It was the thought of seeing my mom that gave me the additional strength. She'd always only heard about my marathon finishes, but now she'd see it with her own eyes.

Andrea was taking my mom and Jaron on a roller-coaster ride. I don't think they were ready for a super spectator experience. That is, one that makes signs, studies the course map for optimal viewing positions, and has prepared race chants for runners. My mother, always a fan of sporting events since she had been young, was accustomed to finding her seat, sitting in it, and only moving to applaud or rebuke participants or refill snacks. But following a pony in this race required you to navigate geography, understand time and distance, and be able to run a 5K yourself. She was so excited the first time she saw me. "Go, son!" she roared like a lioness cheering on one of her cherished cubs. Then they went to lunch—hey, you burn a lot of calories cheering under the scorching hot sun. Mom must've figured they were done until the finish line, because by the fourth time they saw me, her lioness yowls were more like the meow of an ordinary house cat. "What time are you going to be done?" she asked. "Because Andrea has *me* running a marathon all over Chicago too!"

Jaron was still full of energy. He was only eleven at the time, so he was full of zest. As the runners passed him, he slapped high-fives, gave affirmations of their efforts, and let the runners know he was there to support them. I wanted him to witness this race. I only imagined what he might be able to accomplish if he started running marathons earlier than Uncle Jr. and I.

When I crossed the finish line, I felt the heat creep into my veins. My desire to put on a good show for my mom shouldn't have dictated how I approached the race, but it did. I could barely walk. I sat on the curb and waited for my family to arrive. I texted Cathy to see how she was doing.

I have a long way to go. I passed out for fifteen minutes because of the heat, and now I'm walking the last 5K, she texted back.

I sent her my prayers, and I hoped she made it okay as we went back to the hotel to change.

About an hour later, Mom, Andrea, Jaron, Cathy, and I met at Firecakes Donuts. Cathy vividly recalled her out-of-body experience. "I passed out at the twenty-one-mile marker. Slept for thirty minutes, was awakened by spectators and runners thinking I needed medical attention, got up, and finished the race."

I couldn't help but think about what I would have done if heat exhaustion had caused me to pass out, only to awaken with nearly five more miles to go. "I would've had to tap out," I said firmly.

The danger that the heat brings to marathoners is real. Runners have been rushed to the hospital, and some have even died because of it. Nevertheless, I was a marathon finisher in New York City, Boston, Berlin, and Chicago. My thoughts on eating healthy meals and regularly exercising helped fortify me serving as a health role model for my community, and I was well on my way to the marines. Okay, maybe not quite the marines, but the Marine Corps Marathon.

Chapter 16

The Few and the Proud.

In 1993, I was starting my senior year of high school at Cass Technical and hadn't confirmed where I was attending college. My school, an elite prep academy, had a 96 percent graduation rate, and many of my classmates were already sporting sweatshirts and T-shirts of their schools for bragging rights. I, however, had been secretly tossing my acceptance letters in the trash, preparing myself for all the covert operations I'd be part of in the US Marine Corps. My plan was four years in the marines, and I would become the Black 007. I'd been practicing my introduction all summer. "What's your name?" someone would ask. "Moore . . . Charles Moore," I'd respond casually and confidently.

When I got up to courage to tell my mom, I wasn't exactly old enough to make my own decision. At seventeen, I still needed Mom and Dad to sign off on my mission. How would I nab an international terrorist while in a tuxedo if I couldn't even legally enter the casino he's playing in? I should've known I'd be doomed. The Marine Corps recruiter who had sold me described scenes in *Live and Let Die*, *The Man with the Golden Gun*, *The Spy Who Loved Me*, *Moonraker*, *For Your Eyes Only*, *Octopussy*, and *A View to a Kill* as if I were the Moore following up for Roger. He stopped by my house to chat with my parents. He didn't bring the brown manilla envelope with my passport, gun, cash, and instructions, just a cheap attaché case with papers for my mother to sign away her firstborn into military duty.

"Do you really want to do this?" Mom asked with tears already rolling down her cheeks.

"Yes, I do, Mom," I replied with unwavering confidence. But deep inside me, I knew at that moment I would not be going to the marines. There was one person in the world whom I hated to disappoint, and that was Cheryl Lynn Moore.

My dad looked at her and never broke into the smile bubbling up under the surface. "You know he'll never do it. That boy hates getting up early," he said with a smirk, although he'd tell me later that he thought that I just might do it.

As she was signing the paperwork, I couldn't help but think of all the prisoners I'd be saving, the bombs I'd be dismantling, and the champagne I'd be drinking in bars of exotic cities like Baden-Baden, Volgograd, or Podgorica.

I never made it to the marines. During the time between my parents signing me over and me actually going to basic training, I decided I'd prove my dad correct and back out. Never wanting to fall short of my dreams, I ended up a Spartan in East Lansing. But I couldn't help but think of what would've been when I got a lottery entry into the Marine Corps Marathon. The event is the fourth-largest marathon in the United States, with thirty thousand runners. It would be my second time running in Washington, DC.

My spirits were high at the start of this race. I kept thinking about all the ones I'd already finished, so the challenges of this race worried me very little. True, it's still a marathon, but my courage and drive were at their peak. I felt so confident. Confidence is built from experiencing and conquering the challenges and fears you face in life. My career as a marathoner was already in the double digits—and I had finished every race without any major injuries. My main goal was always to finish injury-free.

Before the start, I went through the same routine as for every other race. *After this will be a grand celebration,* I thought. Because I always felt like I'd celebrate hard after a marathon, but, I'd be too exhausted to think about a celebration.

"How many more of these are you doing again?" Andrea asked. She was worried. Every time she watched me tape up my body and plaster my hips, knees, and ankles like an Egyptian mummy, she wondered whether someday one of those limbs would break the tape and burst into flames.

"Two after this: New York and Philly."

We were staying at the Ritz-Carlton in Arlington, Virginia, so it was easy to reach the start, which was just around the corner near the Pentagon. *The Pentagon would probably be where I would've been reporting to headquarters as the Black 007,* I thought.

The beginning of the race seemed to drag, and then suddenly, I was in Georgetown. This neighborhood was pristine; it reminded me of Ann Arbor, Michigan. I checked my Garmin watch for the time and distance, and realized I had only gone five miles. I'd been waiting for a runner to tap me on the shoulder and slip me instructions for my next secret mission all morning. It never happened. When reality set in that I wasn't replacing Daniel Craig as the fictional secret agent, I also realized I was in one of the more boring cities in which to race. The Rock 'n' Roll Running Series marathon in DC seemed to skip all the monuments, maybe to keep the runners' attention on the music, while this event placed all the monuments at our heels. I must admit, none of it moved me until we got to Potomac Parkway, where the tree-lined streets and stone-covered bridges seemed to incrementally increase my adenosine triphosphate, those muscle cells that add energy and give a second wind.

By mile ten, I had passed the Kennedy Center, the Theodore Roosevelt Bridge, and the Lincoln Memorial as easily as I pass on adding milk and sugar to my coffee. None of it drew my interest. Charles Bukowski hated holidays, English accents, and the color orange; I, on the other hand, also have a strong distaste for politicians and enormous landmarks dedicated to them.

Around the halfway mark, my emotions changed. We were running along the Potomac River, and I was surprised to reach the "wear blue" Mile. Either side was lined with photographs of fallen service members and decorated with American flags. All the jokes about me "dodging" the marines started to remind me of what could have happened if I had gone into the corps.

Almost as painful as watching *Marathon: The Patriots Day Bombing* was gazing at the images of real marines, the men and women who didn't make it back home. The patriotism was on the level of Boston. The incitement was eye-opening. Looking around, I noticed all the proud runners draped in full military garb. The runners in uniforms, the flags, the symbolic patches of excellence on their shoulders and chests. It was like Disney, except they weren't in costume, and their expressions were stoic, solemn, and reverent. Jaron could be running this marathon one day, passing my likeness—if I had died while in the marines years ago.

Despite my emotions during the "wear blue" Mile, around mile fourteen, I maintained a spotted viewpoint of the elitism held by marines. Those famous words *semper fidelis* and the motto, "The few, the proud" had held true since its inception.

In 1775, before the United States was an independent country, a dozen Black men served in the newly formed Marine Corps. They fought valiantly, and yet at the end of the American Revolution, as the country for which they bled took shape, heinous discrimination took root. It would be more than 150 years until the corps accepted another Black man.

In 1942, wary of disunity, the US Government ordered the Marine Corps to recruit Black men. Military leaders, including the then-commandant of the corps, resisted the move, but in no time at all, there were nine hundred recruits on their way to North Carolina—to Montford Point.

Constructed only a jog away from Camp Lejeune—the state-of-the-art Whites-only camp for marine recruits—Montford Point became the training ground for thousands of Black marines during the Second World War. After the initial recruitment class, Black marines even took over instruction duties from their White counterparts.

It was a key moment in American history: the US Marine Corps, one of the most elite fighting forces ever assembled, became a desegregated organization in a country that, in many places and in many ways, remained segregated, revealing a little more of "the arc of the moral universe," in the words of Dr. Martin Luther King.

In 2006, sixty years after the first recruits entered their training at Montford Point, approximately 20 percent of all marines were Black, despite Black people making up only 12.4 percent of the US population. These marines carry on the tradition that those nine hundred pioneers began.

^^^

Today was the first time I had a visual race day reminder that only the few and the proud get to finish a marathon, much less the Marine Corps Marathon. By mile seventeen, unarmed guards stood near the gauntlet, (that spot where if you must reach within a certain time), checking their watches for the cutoff time by which a runner would be diverted to another course. By mile twenty, a second crew would check if runners were able to beat the bridge (the other cutoff spot). Around three miles later, a third crew would check if you had made it through the Crystal City gauntlet before the specified cutoff time. The alternate course would have mile markers in case the runners wanted to continue their 26.2-mile jog for personal gratification. However, according to the race's website, these individuals would not be recognized as official finishers. I was proud to complete this race as an official finisher. Upon researching famous finishers of the Marine Corps Marathon, I was pleased to discover several notable names. Kevin Blackistone, a professor and sports journalist of ESPN fame. Supreme Court Justice Clarence Thomas. Former Washington, DC, Mayor Adrian Fenty. And even the queen of media, Oprah Winfrey.

As a Black marathoner, I was standing on the shoulders of giants. Of course, these brilliant names hadn't embarked on the ambitious multi-marathon journey I had laid out for myself. But their distinction on and off the racecourse provided me with a boost and a way forward.

Celebrating my finish at the marathon, a quote from Winfrey came to mind: "Doing the best at this moment puts you in the best place for the next moment." Wise words indeed. Next stop: the New York City Marathon.

Chapter 17

Seven Feet Tall.

November 5 came like it was Easter, Thanksgiving, and Christmas all rolled into one. It always felt like a special holiday in general when Mom was in town, but this time it was her birthday. She never makes a big deal about her birthdays, but she was happy to be in New York City visiting both her sons. And today was the anniversary of my entrance into the running world.

That day, she sat in my living room, watched me get into my battle gear, and pumped me up with everything she planned to say to Uncle Jr. The TV couldn't drown out her roars. "You're going to crush your uncle Jr.'s time this year!" I had already beat his time in other races, but for her, it had to be the same racecourse. And it was personal.

I had been texting all morning with Anca, another marathoner I had befriended a few months ago. She, like Cathy, had run over five New York City marathons, along with a few other cities. We had planned to meet at the ferry and start the race together. *I'll be leaving in ten minutes. Taking a taxi,* I typed.

It was my second time running this course—cruising down the West Side Highway headed to South Ferry, it seemed totally routine. I met Anca, and we were each crushing a banana filled with potassium, magnesium, and calcium to gain an extra morning burst of energy. Not to mention, it was great for cramped muscle relief. This wasn't our first rodeo. The ferry ride was easy, and after a short bus trip, we were at race central. Race central is like a dystopian carnival or a complex maze with a timer. It's only missing farm animals and circus games. "They certainly know how to manage fifty-five thousand runners," I whispered to Anca.

Before you get to the starting line, you have to sort through the five waves—each with six corrals and three start times organized by color. I was in the Green Corral C, Wave 3, and we'd be starting at 10:40 a.m., an hour after the first wave and fifty minutes before the last. Faster runners go out first. And rightfully so; all Keflezighi needs is to spend the entire race dodging runners finishing four or five hours slower than he does.

I ran into James Lu, whom I always get a photo with every time I see him. If you run enough NYRR races, you're bound to bump into James. He started running in his fifties after his wife passed away. By sixty, he was crossing the finish line at his first New York City Marathon. By the time I met him, he'd already bounced through almost twenty NYC marathons and countless local races of shorter distances. You'll know it's him because he always wears a headband with the Japanese flag and runs with the flag of Japan, his five-foot-tall stature dwarfed by the length of his beard and the size of his smile. He just might be the friendliest runner I've ever met.

At the starting line, I looked around for signs of a diverse running field. I was wrong. I gazed across the field of athletes, the faces of the four- and five-hour-paced runners colored with excitement. I couldn't help but think, *These are my peers.* I panned the starting line with my camera, taking in hundreds of runners in front of me and hundreds more behind me. I saw two other Black runners. "I guess there's three of us," I said to myself.

"Did you make a new playlist?" Anca asked. "I got some music that will really get me going this time."

She had already run the event a handful of times, and it was going to be a walk in the park for her. "I'm starting off with my 2016 playlist and plan to divert to some random songs in the middle," I said.

The gun went off. We were on our way!

I watched Anca glide across the Verrazzano-Narrows Bridge and thought, *I need to work on my form.* I watched all the other runners and passed a few. Some blew by me like their human drag reduction system had kicked in. I never worried about who ran faster or slower; I always tried to run my own race. There were more than fifty thousand runners today. *The only one that matters is me,* I told myself. I constantly talked over the music in my head, reminding myself why I was there and what I was going for. Did I know where I was going? Had my "why" changed? My phone buzzed with a new message. It was my mother reminding me I was under strict orders to beat a 5:05 time. So every second counted. *You got this,* she encouraged me.

My uncle Jr. had always been one of my heroes growing up. We spent a lot of time together because we were both into watching basketball, football, and baseball. We went to dozens of Detroit Tigers games every season, and he often indulged my childhood joy by waiting for the players to come out to give autographs. When I switched from collecting Garbage Pail Kids to more lucrative sports cards, he also sharpened my negotiation skills by trading with me. He was relentless. It was my first taste of using statistics to understand markets. "Past performance is no guarantee of future results," he'd say to me when referring to a star player who went bust the following season. In fact, he seemed to always see it coming before it happened. By the time he was done teaching me those lessons in strategy, I became a feared card-trading magnate at school.

By the time Uncle Jr. started running in the late nineties, I had moved to East Lansing and he to Atlanta. So I knew little of his journey until I started mine. By 2015, when I began my quest to break the finish-line tape, I was texting him every now and then seeking tips. He was my only reference for a Black male who ran marathons.

Uncle Jr. would tell me:

I started running around March 1998 to lose weight. I was about 236 pounds at the time, and my goal was to get down to 165 pounds. I was thirty-eight years old at the time, and I had never run seriously at all. Prior to that, I was surprised how easy it was for me and how much I loved it. I kept a journal and tracked my miles run, my time, and the course. After a while, I started buying running shoes every several months and started entering 5K and 10K races. I loved it. I love the fact that running was therapeutic for me. I could solve all my problems in a seventy-five-minute run. It was exhilarating!

I had run several 5K and 10K races in Detroit and an 8K race in Atlanta, Georgia, and I wanted to test myself in a longer race. My daily runs were generally ten to fifteen miles with an occasional seventeen- to twenty-mile run, so I figured I could run six more miles with no problem. So I entered the 2000 NYC Marathon lottery, not really expecting to get in. NYC runners were given a higher priority in getting in, and therefore, many outsiders or nonresidents were turned away unless you were an elite runner. Lo and behold, I received an email notifying me that I was among the lucky few—relatively speaking—to receive a race number.

My best friend lived in Hell's Kitchen at the time, so I contacted him and made plans to stay there for ten days. He was newly graduated from the Culinary Institute of America, so he put his chef skills to work and made sure I carbo-loaded leading up to race day. He worked at Mario Batali's Babbo Ristorante at the time. My friend introduced me to Batali, and he brought out some Italian tapas with just enough pasta—and a glass of wine—on the eve of race day.

The morning of the race, I was super excited. We got up around 4 a.m., I had a half cup of coffee, a half a banana, and some granola. We headed out to the bus that would take me from Manhattan over into Staten Island. I wore several layers of clothing for the chilly weather, expecting to unpeel them deeper into the race. I looked around me at my fellow runners and was never so excited to start a race. The New York City Marathon.

The gun sounded, and we all headed out on the Verrazzano-Narrows Bridge. What I remember most was the lovely view and the beautiful sea of people in front of me and behind me. I had run a quarter of a mile at a safe jog with others when I noticed a round, black wire object in front of me. I tried my best to avoid it, but I noticed it too late and my foot got tangled in it. I fell face down on the bridge, and as I fell, all I could think about was the front of the *New York Daily News* with the headline: "Atlanta, Georgia, Man Trampled by Fellow Runners in the NY City Marathon." But no sooner had I fell, runners on both sides of me picked me up immediately before any damage was done. My knees were burning, but the embarrassment was worst. It wasn't until I was about three miles into the race that I noticed my knees were scratched and blood running down my left leg. I was fine until I saw that. I decided I would not let that destroy everything I had worked for, and so I soldiered on. I didn't feel any distress until I hit the twenty-one-mile mark. I have since learned that's usually the place most novices start feeling it. I live and run by the motto "Pain is inevitable. Suffering is optional," and that was certainly the case here.

I finished the race in a time of 5:05. Not a fast time by any measure, but I felt a real sense of accomplishment and one I will never forget. I've run other distances since then but have not completed another marathon. At age sixty-two, my love for running has not diminished at all. I still run four to five days a week—sometimes more, sometimes less. I will likely continue to run until my legs give out.

That's my November 5, 2000, NYC Marathon experience.

^^^

By the time I reached mile twenty-three, it was apparent that this was going to be a photo finish. Looking at my splits, I was only drifting about a minute per mile. Later, I found out that my mother and Uncle Jr. were trading jabs—again. No sucker punches, just good, clean, wholesome sibling rivalry, with me caught in the middle. Except my mom was right there, on her birthday, bouncing through all five boroughs, cheering even more than the superfans.

As I approached the final mile, I felt good and thought I'd beat Uncle Jr.'s time by a few minutes. I joined the text thread between my mom and Uncle Jr., and boasted, "I'm going to have a four in front of my time." I gazed into the stands at the VIP section and saw my crew. Knowing Mom was not quite up for a Chicago repeat, I ponied up for the stadium seating at the finish. The stands mimic high school bleachers, enclosing the final four hundred meters, one set on each side, so spectators can sit and watch all the finishers. The feeling I got as I ran by and waved frightened me. My first thought was, *The families at the Boston Marathon bombing were waving at their loved one when disaster struck.* I crossed my heart and prayed my family and friends would see one another soon after the day's race was over.

And as I crossed the finish line, I checked my watch. It read 4:59. I'd just beat the GOAT.

^^^

At home, my celebration ended, and now it was all about celebrating my mom's special day. Keeping with tradition, I ordered everyone steaks from Keens Steakhouse. DJ brought a birthday cake. Mom, who never drinks, had a glass of Armand de Brignac—a French champagne owned by Möet Hennessy Diageo and Mr. Shawn Carter, aka Jay-Z. It was a touch of luxury and decadence as a treat for her and well worth enjoying on this joyous occasion.

Also keeping with tradition, I took off work the next day. My mom and I walked the neighborhood, her in her 2016 marathon sweater and me with my 2017 marathon medal. Three blocks away, we ran into the Admiral: NBA champion and former San Antonio Spurs center David Robinson. How do you miss a guy *literally* seven feet tall? He was one of my uncle Jr.'s favorite basketball players back in the nineties and early aughts. "Can we get a picture?" He smiled and said, "Of course."

I, too, felt like a champion that day. Not for having encountered a larger-than-life champion, but for living up to the promise I had made to myself to be a (self)-competing Black marathon runner, inspiring not only the next generation of Black marathoners, but those closest to me as well. I could do anything I set my mind to. Next stop—race time in Philadelphia.

Chapter 18

The Nod.

When I returned to Philadelphia after the first marathon, I couldn't stop thinking about the nod. I couldn't help but contemplate a few questions. Why Philly? Why me? Or were all Black runners getting the nod from other Black runners? Why hasn't anything changed?

The majority of America may not comprehend it or even know why it exists, this subtle raising or lowering of the head, giving affirmation and acknowledgment that the two of us are here. Usually done between Black men, it is a method to understand a few things: "I see you." "You're safe." "I have your back." Or "Awesome, I'm not the only one."

Why couldn't we just celebrate like everyone else and clink glasses and toast; cheers, *salud*, or mazel tov? We do that too. But so does almost everyone else. We needed something that was for us, by us. We needed something to secretly signal to the other, a nod to say, "You are seen by me," even if no one else sees you.

Running may seem simple. It is, to an extent. Yet there are risks involved—especially for Black runners, many of which don't exist for White athletes. Black runners may be hyperfocused on their surroundings during distance runs, making a conscious, sometimes exhausting effort to overcome racial stereotypes, blend in, and put others at ease. *Runner's World* explains that to prevent potential conflict, Black runners may wear T-shirts from their university, as if to say, "I went to college. Don't shoot me." They may exclusively run in well-lit areas, waving and smiling at passersby as if to say, "I come in peace." Naturally, this can be exhausting. Few White runners understand, pushing Black athletes into further isolation. Or to just not run at all.

I struck up a conversation at the expo in Philly with a White gentleman from the Chestnut Hill area of the city. He boasted, "Running outdoors makes me feel so free, and I get to breathe the fresh air in the park and see all the green."

"Yeah," I replied, "but I only run outside on race day."

He gave me a quizzical look, but I couldn't exactly explain my reasoning either. After reading about Black runners, I wasn't exactly sure anymore. Was it because I still had a recurring Equinox gym bill on my credit card? Or was my subconscious mind telling me I was safer running indoors?

So I started researching topics like "health," "Black," and "running" online. I had no clue there were organizations focused on the health and well-being of Black distance runners. Many such athletes, especially in long-distance running, advocate for more diversity and more community resources. Organizations in support of Black distance running are integral to this initiative— and one man, in particular, is intent on making it happen. Tony Reed, celebrated distance runner and cofounder of the National

Black Marathoners' Association (NBMA), holds an impressive résumé. A member of the National Black Distance Running Hall of Fame, his accomplishments include being the first Black person to have finished a marathon on all seven continents. Clearly, Reed invests a great deal in his own running career. His priority, however, is extolling the virtues of the NBMA to other distance runners and stakeholders—and sharing the history of Black American distance running with the general public.

The country's oldest, largest nonprofit organization of Black American distance runners, the NBMA is open to everyone, regardless of running ability or marathon experience. The organization's website notes that 40 percent of its members have yet to complete a marathon and that many prefer walking to running. Ultimately, the NBMA strives to encourage members of the Black community to work toward a healthy lifestyle by way of distance running and walking. It allows runners to meet in large groups at marathons across the country. And while the organization aims to celebrate the accomplishments of Black American runners, its most critical aim is to make running more *accessible*. The NBMA offers scholarships to high school-age Black distance runners; it has awarded more than $50,000 in funds to date. I hadn't seen them at any of the races I had participated in, but I now had my eyes open for a T-shirt or a sign.

Philadelphia has always been a city I have loved. But when I couldn't make those cherished weekend trips to Philly, I missed the realness of the dark and gloomy emptiness of streets like Lehigh Avenue and West Oakdale Street. "In anxiety, one feels uncanny," Heidegger said. Perhaps I couldn't imagine the prejudice that existed in the late 1800s against Jews, Blacks, and Italians in South Philly.

Dilapidated neighborhoods are not ideal places to train for a marathon. Access to running communities and resources in a healthy living space are integral. This is just one of the reasons why organizations for Black distance runners are so impactful. According to "The State of Obesity: Better Policies for a Healthier America," Black American adults are 1.5 times more likely to be obese than their White counterparts. Similarly, more than 75 percent of Black Americans are overweight or obese compared with just 67.2 percent of White Americans; the mortality rates from heart disease and stroke are almost double among Blacks. In Philly, over 40 percent of the Black community self-reported as obese. This paints a shocking picture of the health disparities at play—making organizations for Black distance runners imperative to improving health outcomes.

It was two weeks prior in New York City where I first started to see shirts that read *Black Men Run* and *Black Girls RUN!* In Philadelphia, with my eyes wide open, nodding every time I saw a fellow Black runner, I would cheer even louder when I saw these groups.

First, there was a large group of women bearing T-shirts, hats, and bags emblazoned with slogans. They cheered for everyone. But when I came running by, they roared. "Go get 'em!" one lady yelled.

"I'm trying," I panted a little while in midstride. I really was trying. I was there to try to understand the landscape of marathoning and who gets to participate.

By the fifth mile, I ran across the men. Dressed in all black, their group's name was in bold, red letters: Black Men Run. I high-fived one guy. Another guy yelled, "I see you, brother!" And then two guys, in near-perfect unison; their faces stoic and shielding their pride, gave me the nod. I understood now. These were Black fraternities and sororities. The groups may have had their respective spots, but their makeup was mixed. Men, women, Latinx, and White people, all showing support.

While an individual sport, distance running is rooted in camaraderie and community. People might train together, run races in groups, and ask for advice or guidance (or simply someone to confide in). Both men and women benefit from joining organizations catering exclusively to Black distance running, which is precisely where nonprofits like Black Men Run and Black Girls RUN! come in.

The home page of the former's website reads *Brotherhood, Unity, Health* because Black Men Run strives not to create future Olympians (though all are welcome), but to inspire general fitness and a culture of running. The team behind the organization believes that running and jogging can help mitigate the health and fitness disparities between White and Black Americans, all while encouraging African American men to get out and move their bodies. The organization emphasizes that as the research is homing in on the physical benefits of distance running, the sport can also improve mental sharpness, boost confidence, and relieve stress—elements that will further serve the Black male community.

Cofounded by distance runners Jason L. Russell and Edward Walton, the organization's leaders cite peace, clarity, and community as just some of the reasons they get out and run most days. But overall, the men's goal is to cultivate a group of Black men dedicated to living and promoting a healthy lifestyle.

Similarly, Toni Carey, who founded Black Girls RUN! in 2009, set out to overturn the misconception that Black women

don't run. And while she recognizes the obesity epidemic facing
the Black community, she rightfully believes encouragement,
resources, and access to a community of runners can help. Like
Black Men Run, Black Girls RUN! helps Black women prioritize
healthy living in their daily routines. Carey hopes that through
running, education, and social connection she can help lower
the percentage of women experiencing chronic disease and
weight challenges linked to a sedentary lifestyle. People from
anywhere in the world can join the community, subscribe to
the newsletter, invest in the recommended gear, and digitally
connect with other members. The community's resources are
expansive, ranging from meetups and ambassador programs to
tips on how best to offset the cost of inflation while building a
running practice.

^^^

My head and heart felt so heavy, like I was carrying an extra
fifty pounds. My mind raced thinking about these groups, this
community, and the entire running culture. I almost didn't notice
how windy it was on Kelly Drive. I didn't know which was moving
faster: visions of the logos from these groups in my head or my
feet trying to complete this marathon. I checked my watch, and
it appeared I was making good time. Mile eighteen going into
nineteen was a breeze.

At least that's what I told myself. I texted Andrea about fifteen
minutes prior to tell her I was having *literal* stomach cramps.
This from a guy who always knows the locations of the five-star
hotels because they have the cleanest bathrooms. I despise using
public restroom facilities so much that just thinking about it
ruins my day. I always joke, "The day I have to use a Porta Potty

is the day I DNF because I *will* tap out."

Can't get a DNF, can't get a DNF, I repeated over and over in my head. And I suddenly realized, whatever I was doing to try to distract myself wasn't going to last 7.2 miles. Once I got to mile twenty, I called Andrea. "If I used the latrine in the middle, it'll be the one least used . . . right?"

I heard a pause and then a mischievous giggle. "It's like *The Price Is Right*, Charles. What's behind door number four?" she joked.

I didn't know what to feel. I felt like I could cry—but I needed that precious liquid to stay hydrated. So I didn't. I wanted to yell. But nothing came out. I was too close to give up, and I felt fine otherwise.

I whipped out my phone. I realized the finish line was closer than the restroom at the Four Seasons Hotel. There would be no one who would comprehend, understand, or have sympathy for me if I chose to quit—including me. I kept running. But the rumble in my stomach felt like each step was only bringing me closer to a volcanic eruption.

I saw a Starbucks. I ran in. The line for the restroom was full of spectators; at least I knew there were no runners. I had no time to waste. "I'm running the marathon, and I need to go to the bathroom," I declared like an announcer at a Flyers game.

The entire line parted like I was Moses, and I was promoted to the front of the line.

Later, Andrea called to check on me. "Are you okay?"

I gave her the same pause she had dished out earlier. "I am one Tough Mudder!"

Laughing, she sensed I was back on course. She and her mom were just finishing afternoon tea. It was her mom's third race, and I was happy she was there in her hometown. My mother-in-law, born and raised in Philly, was as street smart as they come. I remember waiting for her at Penn Station when she'd make the trek via Amtrak: her back against the wall, eyes scanning the station, hand tightly clinching her handbag. You weren't going to finesse Arline; you'd have to look her dead in the eyes if you were going to snatch her bag. Andrea, raised in Wilmington, Delaware, had never had to watch out for wolves.

Once, Andrea and I were in Beijing, China, and a savvy rickshaw driver spotted fresh, easy prey: us. It was about 108 degrees, easy. "Let's just take this rickshaw to the subway," Andrea groaned.

But I had a bad feeling about him. The entire ride, I was watching Google Maps. "You're going the wrong way," I repeated over and over.

He ignored me, with Andrea chiming in, "Don't be so coupe de ville." Thinking I was too snobby to get on a rickshaw.

When we finally arrived, still a quarter of a mile from the subway stop and having taken twenty minutes longer than expected, he demanded $300.

I turned to Andrea to remind her, "It's your mother that's from Philly." I threw him five bucks and we left.

Arline picked the restaurant, one of her favorites, Dante & Luigi's, a fine Italian establishment. Post-marathon dinners were often spent reminiscing about the race, the experience, and of course, the medal. It was fitting that this medal was literally a miniature version of the Liberty Bell. I tried to toll it, but it didn't make a sound. Silent, like the nod all those runners gave me a year ago and today.

What was so different about Philly? What about the culture, the community, and their experiences led them to show me they saw me? The City of Brotherly Love really left a mark on me. I finished the race setting a personal record. That my time meant nothing to me was an understatement. I thought only about whether I had accomplished what I had set out to. I hadn't. At this point, I was two marathons away from completing the six Abbott World Marathon Majors. Only London and Tokyo remained.

Chapter 19

Heat Wave.

It's crazy to think that my first time in Miami was 2016. I'd gone down there with Michael, Alessandro, Max, and a few other guys for Michael's bachelor party. We had a blast. Even when I informed them that we couldn't be in such a culturally rich city without visiting the Pérez Art Museum Miami and the Rubell Museum, they protested mildly, but were all blown away by the collections. I'd return later that year to attend Art Basel Miami Beach for the first of many times. By January 2018, I was a Dade County pro.

As unavoidable as it may seem, I was not expecting eighty degrees. Or at least, I was hoping it wouldn't be eighty degrees. Today would be a first. For the first time, the entire expo chitter-chatter was about the impact that the heat would have on the weekend's race. With climate change comes a spike in global heat waves. Paired with longer, hotter summers in many regions, the gradual rise in temperature—and the increase in long-term heat waves—places immense strain on the planet.

Hydration was my complete focus in the weeks before the race. I amped up my Nuun intake and added Hammer's Endurolytes. We in the Black community were always told that high-sodium diets were one of the primary causes of high blood pressure, heart disease, and stroke—all ailments radically plaguing African Americans. I had learned in recent months that high sodium, at least if you are an endurance athlete exercising in heat-stress environments, is your best friend. I wasn't popping them like gummy bears, but I chose to take half the recommended pill count just in case. Knowing my body's reaction to extreme heat, though, it was safe to assume that I needed to balance my engine's cooling system.

In addition to the environmental issues resulting from these heat waves, extreme heat presents a number of physical risks to adults. Exposure to heat waves is problematic for even the healthiest of people, as our bodies are meant to maintain a constant core temperature of ninety-eight degrees. That's why ideal temperatures during a marathon are in the forties and fifties.

In simple terms, health issues begin to occur when an adult's core body temperature gets too hot, especially while performing high-intensity exercise like distance running. The organs and enzymes may shut down in these cases, and kidney issues, heart problems, and even brain damage may occur in the long term. Generally, race organizers plan their events during a time of year when they see favorable temperatures in their city. For example, New York City is in the fall and Boston is in spring, so it's natural that Miami would host theirs in the winter. Experts say there is a limit to human tolerance for heat and cold, yet individuals should understand their own body and how it reacts to certain temperatures. I know that increased exposure to the sun and temperatures above eighty are not friendly to me. Those factors sound like going for a casual stroll in Death Valley, California.

I vividly remember my first time going to Miami. In 2016, Michael asked me to help plan his bachelor party, which would include Max, Alessandro, and Ryan. Michael's brother would join us later, but only for our final steak dinner. I picked Miami for two reasons: it was easy for everyone to get to, and I had never been there. During all my years living in New York City, I had heard all my friends talk about flying south for the winter or going to Miami because it was a quick getaway, but I had never made the trip.

We went to the beach, shopped in the Design District, visited a museum or two, and had plenty of casual strolls up and down Ocean Drive. We had all initially met in Rome, so of course nothing compares with walking into a random church and seeing an original Caravaggio painting or a five-hundred-year-old sculpture by Michelangelo, debating during your jaunts through the city who had worked the chisel better: Bernini or Borromini. But Miami did have the collections of the Rubell Museum, de la Cruz, and Pérez. We would certainly enjoy a Kusama installation or a Koons painting. We all loved art, and that was a major highlight. "This was great, Charles, but when are we getting drinks?" Ryan teased.

Okay, so we all liked art, but we were supposed to be celebrating our good friend getting married.

The thing I remember the most of that five-day weekend is the night we went to the club after a late dinner. When we finally left at 9 a.m., I was dragging them out the door, only to see that there was still a line to get in. The next day we were totally energized—(not!)—exhausting our pointer fingers in the air poolside, requesting more water to rehydrate after the evening before festivities.

^^^

The race started promptly at six in the morning. It was ideal to begin early, as you want to be finished before the hottest part of the day in the afternoon. "Be careful with the wind," one runner said to me on my left.

From my right, another chimed in, "The wind will trick you into thinking it is cooler than it is."

I glanced up in front of me, and someone in official gear was unfurling a teardrop-shaped event alert banner: from moderate to high. Up to this point, green banners had been hung proudly at almost every race I had run, like college automobile decals, marking conditions as good for running. I've even seen the yellow ones, boldly stating the conditions were less than ideal, with occasional announcements saying, "Be prepared for worsening conditions." But I had never seen the elusive, raspberry-colored symbol announcing potentially dangerous conditions.

I wasn't nervous, but I did want the group of blabbering runners next to me to lower their voices. All the talk about how nervous they were was influencing me too. I panicked—three walls were closing in on me, and the only way out was to turn around and go back to my hotel. *As if I would quit the race because I was too hot.* Without that fourth wall to box me in, there was no way I'd be losing to the Miami heat without a fight.

As the race started, I got a text from my friend, who called me Mr. Ferrari. Not because I own a Ferrari, but because I ran so many marathons. Her text read, *You can't let a Ferrari overheat.* So I'd better stay hydrated.

The race started in Downtown Miami, immediately hitting the 5K-long MacArthur Causeway straight to South Beach. The runners held their arms up, looking like Winfrey giving away gifts to her audience—"*You* get a marathon medal! *You* get a marathon medal! *Everybody* gets a marathon medal!" We pounded our feet against the six-lane slab of metal as we headed for the beach side of town.

A runner next to me sighed. "Ah, I just love this breeze."

My mind went back to those runners beside me at the start. "Be careful with the wind," I warned her. "It'll fool you into thinking it's cooler than it is out." I felt like Bernie Lootz from the film *The Cooler* raining on everyone's parade.

The bridge is long and picturesque, overlooking the yachts, beachfront properties, and cruise ships. After gobbling up the three-mile bridge, I finally reached the beach side.

Runners' heels clapped the concrete like spectator cheers. As we crossed into the beach side, we encountered men and women dressed as if they had left a disco party—it was just past 9 a.m. The looks on their faces were as dismayed as ours; their nights were ending as our days were just beginning. Partygoers were leaving clubs as we rounded the corner to Ocean Drive.

By this time, I had been to Miami a few times. I had visited only a few weeks ago for an art fair. Miami Beach had been hosting the international art fair, Art Basel, for over a decade by then. Art patrons and galleries across continents attended this event annually, and some of the biggest deals of the year would be made. Visitors could discover the latest trends and the most prominent names among living artists.

While I was in middle school, my mother, the first art collector I knew, carted me around to local fairs and festivals, plucking out paintings and prints to decorate our walls with images that showed her version of the Black experience. I developed my taste for art casually back then but wasn't in love yet. While in college, I'd visit the Detroit Institute of Arts whenever I was back home for the holidays. But when I arrived in New York City in 2005, I was starving for culture. I spent countless hours at the Metropolitan Museum of Art, the Whitney Museum of American Art, and the Museum of Modern Art. My time in Europe had taught me a lesson in the old masters. From 2009 to 2012, I traveled extensively, visiting over fifty museums and learning more about periods, brushstrokes, and biographies.

In 2012, a trip to Boston marked my humble art-collecting beginnings. Upon visiting the Institute of Contemporary Art, I exited through the gift shop and purchased a limited-edition print by Shepard Fairey for $50. I was obsessed with collecting ever since. I devoured books and documentaries on artists. I read market reports and news from online journals. I was really doing something. But it wasn't until 2017, when I met an art adviser, that my life was changed. I no longer collected prints and editions; original paintings and sculptures started to grace my walls. I slowed my acquisitions almost to a halt, buying more selectively than on impulse. Some people travel to Miami to get away from the cold northern winters; I travel to Miami for the heat of the scorching fine art scene.

^^^

The number 81 started to stick in my head. I knew I wasn't going to see Andrea for a while. The race had started too early, and we were staying on the mainland. As I was leaving the beach side, approaching the fluid station on Belle Isle, the heat really started to kick in. If Philly was my personal record, Miami was surely going to be my personal worst. My head felt like it was floating away. The salt left my body through sweat faster than the balls leaving the racquets on Miami tennis courts. I cracked open my pouch only to find my salt sticks had melted. I had dropped my Endurolyte tablets back on mile four. *Don't panic,* I said to myself.

I arrived at the fluid station, and luckily, they had bananas and Gatorade. Major crisis averted, but I had to figure out exactly how much time I had before I'd crash. My ciele cap was barely shielding me from the sun. My lululemon tights were now overheating my legs. But at least my HOKA Clifton 4s made each step feel casual. I like the padding of HOKAs; it feels like you're running with pillows strapped to your feet.

I slowed my pace to a brisk walk and thought about lasting the final sixteen miles. By the time I got to the half-marathon breakaway point, I thought, *Wouldn't it be so great to be done now?* Mental toughness is hard for me to measure, and I'm unsure how it can be taught. All I know is that at every marathon I've run, there wasn't a time where I didn't tell myself, *I'm never doing this again.* In Miami, I must have said it on twenty-six occasions. The back of my neck was burning, sun-damaged. My legs felt like I had snow pants on in the middle of summer. And the pit of my stomach drowned in anxiety, begging for something other than GU Energy Chews and warm water. Righteous men do not run marathons. This was definitely the devil working against me.

When the marathon was done, I felt like I had been auditioning for Ethan Hawke's role in *Training Day.* Denzel Washington had just run me all over the city, and I got a gaudy faux gold medal to prove it. I finished. I didn't know if I wanted to party at Fontainebleau's LIV or chill in Faena Hotel's Tierra Santa Healing House. But I needed a shower. It was only then I remembered that I had forgotten to put on the anti-chafing body-glide cream, and every drop of water that hit my armpits and thighs felt like an attack by bullet ants and warrior wasps.

"What's going on in there?" Andrea asked in response to my moans.

"The water is burning my skin off!"

But this was only the beginning of a heat wave. Next stop was Hotlanta, an integral part of the Dirty South hip-hop scene.

Chapter 20

Panda Bears.

"Welcome to Atlanta, jackin' hammer and vogues," rapped Ludacris on Jermaine Dupri's 2001 album *Instructions*. Unlike Luda, I did not make it to the Waffle House on this trip. However, he should've added the lyrics "Where the sun is especially hot" because that weekend in March 2018, it was approximately thirty degrees warmer than one would hope for a marathon. I was aware of that and expected it for a city nicknamed Hotlanta. But it didn't make it any less shocking to the system to experience that kind of heat while running. This would be my first time returning to Atlanta since I had been in middle school when I had competed in the national tournament for AGLOA.

I felt I knew the city already. My uncle Jr. had lived there for over twenty years, their zoo had panda bears (my favorite animal), and it was considered for a decade or so, around the turn of the new millennium, to be the new Motown. Though none of this was the most pressing thought going through my head; I thought a lot about the people. Especially with historically Black colleges and universities like Spelman and Morehouse, and employers that helped catapult Blacks to the upper middle class like Coca-Cola and Delta Airlines, the Black community financially flourished to achieve the status of affluent in metropolitan Atlanta. I expected to see a large Black crowd at the marathon, running and cheering. To unwind, I ventured to Zoo Atlanta.

Walking through your local zoo, you are unlikely to see a panda bear. Pandas can be seen in only twenty-six zoos across twenty countries. These countries are either in close proximity to China or have well-funded zoological programs. In the United States, there were only four zoos in which you can see a panda; Smithsonian National Zoological Park in Washington, DC, Zoo Atlanta, Memphis Zoo, and San Diego Zoo Wildlife Alliance. That number is dwindling, since even at the time of writing this book the pandas have left San Diego.

There are a few barriers to being lucky enough to have a panda in your zoo. First, China owns all the pandas in the world. They rent them to zoos for up to $1 million, with a $400,000 price tag on keeping any cubs that come from successful mating. Tack on the cost of research and development, the habitat upkeep, and salaries for the zoologists who specialize in giant pandas, and you're in for well over $2 million a year. Impressed yet?

Walking through Zoo Atlanta, I was bewildered because the panda is such a majestic and striking creature to behold. When you stand in its presence, you cannot help but feel the gentleness of its character, the way it plods from bamboo stalk to shaded nest, reveling in the simplicity of its lifestyle, enjoying the tranquility that is its life. I couldn't help but notice the dichotomy of its black-and-white characteristics. The hues weren't separate. They meshed harmoniously as one body.

After the zoo, I popped into the High Museum of Art. Located in the heart of the city, the museum boasts almost 20,000 works of art, spanning multiple periods and regions. As I'm walking up to the museum, I can't help but notice *House III*. The colorful rendition of Lichtenstein's house series is meant to capture the essence of the suburban American home. "Some assembly required, white picket fence sold separately," I said to a stranger walking by. She clearly got my joke. "Yeah, if you're middle class and White," she murmured in response.

When I got inside, I had one thing in mind: find the Kehinde. At the time, Kehinde Wiley was already a household name outside the art community. His portrait of the forty-fourth president of the United States hanging in the National Portrait Gallery cemented him as one of the most important painters of our time. But long before gracing the halls of one of the Smithsonian Institution's most important collections, he was participating in residencies around the globe. One such residency was in Brazil, where Afro-Brazilian men became the focal point of the work he did there. In Brazil, like in many South American countries, being darker-skinned meant you were less than. So when Wiley selected men like Thiago Oliveira do Rosario Rozendo to sit for him, he put them on the world stage. I pondered the idea of what it must feel like to be one of few in Brazil. Like Andrew in London.

I often feel that when I am running a marathon, I can empathize with any panda that may question why there are so few like it anywhere in sight. I have come to expect that the makeup of each marathon I run will look like the makeup of every marathon before it, crowds of White people cheering on the sidelines and a steady flow of White people running on either side of me. A few spots of Black people sprinkled in here and there. Not exactly the coloring of a panda bear. But Atlanta had to be different, right?

Oh, and I wasn't looking for homogeneity—a score of all-Black (or even mostly Black) runners; I'm looking for representation. I'm looking to uplift and to be uplifted by my community. Culture encompasses many things—identification with gender, religious group, spoken language, work group, racial identity, and more. In fact, all of us are a single monoculture in and of ourselves. There will never be another Charles Moore like me, and there will never be another person like you either; we are each uniquely unique.

In marathoning, I felt well represented as a male, as a well-educated person, as a polyglot (English and Italian), and as a music lover—but not so much as a Black man. For I am the metaphorical marathon panda. Can you see it wearing a pair of HOKAs? Can you see white-and-black-striped runners draped in Tracksmith race attire? Can you see us all being its healthiest? It needed not be white with a few black spots on its knees and abdomen. It needed a healthy mix like the pandas at Zoo Atlanta.

Speaking of Atlanta, I had trained hard for this race. I did a few short runs after Miami to stay loose. My uncle Jr. in Atlanta would tell me he ran daily and all about his small group of running buddies he'd meet up with for a light 5K or 10K weekend run. Atlanta was a place where Black people don't visit, they move out here, Jermaine Dupri said. Not unlike my uncle Jr., Atlanta, a place where Black people have regularly taken on positions of power in government and business and the arts; this seemed like it would be the one place where the trend might change. Perhaps there, as nowhere else in America, I might look out at the crowd and see skin that looked like mine.

I was sorely mistaken.

Even in Atlanta, the demographics of marathoning were apparent. It felt just like other marathons in that regard. Though that feeling allowed me to reflect on what Atlanta represented to the Black community.

There is a sense in Atlanta that one can connect with people and build something, that the social and economic constraints and the binds, so pernicious elsewhere, become looser in the face of so much Black excellence, so much Black wealth, and so much Black success. While gentrification in other cities like Chicago and Brooklyn has cast a pall over Black legacies and traditions, the community has thrived there because the system is set up in such a way that there is support and resources. In Atlanta, our youth can count on education, but more importantly, they can count on role models and bustling industries headed by Black men and women who were educated in that fine city.

As I was preparing to start the Atlanta Marathon, all these facts were on my mind. At the time, they seemed disconnected from my visit to Zoo Atlanta. I had done something there that only a fraction of American zoos would enable me to do: view pandas in their lush and spacious pen.

One is never alone among the pandas. This is true in two distinct senses. The first is that because the panda is such a singularly popular animal to see, the crowd is constant. All around you, locals and tourists are standing shoulder to shoulder. We all took in the pandas with the awe that this herbivorous bear commands. The second sense in which one is never alone among the pandas is the tranquility that characterizes the animals. Even their eyes seem to open and close with all the grace of a runner.

^ ^ ^

After I left Zoo Atlanta, the pandas came with me in spirit, and I remembered them as I lined up at the starting line. I thought about them, their rarity, and connected them to my own rareness there on the course. I connected them to what that rarity meant, not just to me but to Black children: When they saw a panda bear, like seeing adults who looked like them at their local marathon, did it feel out of place—or did it feel special? Did it feel like an anomaly—or like a beautiful moment worth cherishing and worth claiming again and again?

Black Men Run, one of the most important organizations dedicated to promoting running among Black men, started in Atlanta. Their initiatives seek to normalize marathoning among the Black community. Their presence was felt, but only in small spots.

On that course, most of my attention at the time was on the race in front of me. As I took off from the starting line, I thought not about stresses or anxieties. Rather, I was able to process them while running and work my way through them. My breath crushed together inside my lungs, my cheeks burned from all the sweat that seeped from my body, and I steadfastly refused to slow down, however much my feet cried out for me to do so.

As I ran past Martin Luther King, Jr. National Historical Park and on to the Jimmy Carter Presidential Library & Museum, it was just the course and me, the thousands of other runners there another part of the backdrop. This is marathoning, a sport that tempts you to let go of that steady stream of words and ideas that moves relentlessly through your mind otherwise. That day I welcomed such a respite, surprised as I was that, although the Atlanta Marathon was in Atlanta, it was still much more firmly in the society of all marathons, a society intertwined in a picturesque tapestry of colors.

Event alert banners were everywhere, bleeding *Moderate: Use Caution*. The other banners I noticed were the signs held by spectators. One read: *If A Marathon Was Easy, It'd Be Called Your Mother*. Another read: *Go Random Stranger*. My laughter at finally noticing the carefully drawn-out, (somewhat) creatively crafted words plastered on vision boards was what kept me going. I always casually blew by these signs, but something made me open my eyes during this race to read them. Besides, they had gotten up early in the morning to color, day drink, and slur arbitrary versions of the English language for hours on a Sunday. They were the real heroes!

I didn't see a Black Men Run T-shirt until mile twenty. *Finally*, I thought to myself. A group of around a hundred or so men and women were posted along my right side of the course. I slowed my pace to a halt and walked by. "Thank you for coming out today!" I shouted.

"No, bro, thank you for running," one guy responded.

Suddenly, a young lady around thirtyish, wearing a Spelman T-shirt, ran up and said, "Way to go, sir! You got this!" Her energy was electrifying. But I didn't know whether she was about to run with me or slap me a high-five. Either way, I felt charged up.

Black Men Run originated in Atlanta not out of some abstract desire for Black men to run, but as a response to a pivotal question: How do Black Americans find safe spaces in which to run? In an era in which Ahmaud Arbery lost his life looking for just that, this question carries some hefty weight. Although we are still working to answer it in practice, the reality is clear: Black Americans will be safe and comfortable running as more Black Americans start to run, as the group is there to affirm and validate our presence. That corner gave me a strong sense of pride. I no longer felt the need to count the runners or spectators for the rest of the day. All I needed to see was that.

Black affluence in Atlanta, Black presence on the course, and panda bears. A symbol of peace like the marathon itself, the panda inspired me that day to see the marathon as a path that we can run together. It is a solitary animal, but in its fur, I thought while I was gasping for breath somewhere between the first mile and the twenty-sixth, the beauty of togetherness is undeniable.

On marathon courses, from Atlanta to Tokyo and every city in between, we may someday find that value just the same. Humans have so much to learn from the animal kingdom. That day, I learned so much and was even inspired by the majestic panda. Next up was another marathon and a global city that, at the time, also had one of the world's few zoos that boasted a majestic panda: London town.

Chapter 21

Battered Warriors.

And suddenly, there was an abrupt stop. The next four weeks after Atlanta, my training stopped. I had no clue as to why I didn't move. My knees were fine. My heart pumped normally. And psychologically, I felt incredibly accomplished. But something felt different. You'd think I'd be just peachy after finishing an Atlanta marathon in the great state of Georgia, the Peach State, but no.

It seemed my muscles burned every day. My calves were especially hot, like I had had a few bites of Carolina Reaper peppers, but the intense burning sensation had skipped my tongue and soft palate, and pooled in my lower legs instead. I thought I had lactic acid buildup, which, apparently, is a result of insufficient oxygen intake during exercise. I waited until two weeks before London to start researching. Most of the articles I read equated the feeling to drinking poison. This felt akin to my experience, but the feeling was supposed to dissipate eventually.

I realized only then that my body was numb all of 2017 from 365 days of adrenaline pumping in my veins. I was crashing. Charles Moore's body was officially on strike, my legs and muscles the strike's ringleaders.

I didn't know what to do. It was the first time I didn't do anything between races. I didn't stretch. I didn't run a single mile. I didn't even lift a ten-pound dumbbell. I went to class, wrote my papers, read, slept, and occasionally ate. I wondered if this was a form of depression. I always felt a slight drop in my spirits after each race. I never wanted to admit it, but the post-marathon blues for me were real. But I'd always register for another race just as soon as my mood came back like a boomerang. I often shifted gears by tapping my small network of running friends. I'd text Anca or Cathy or Matt or Andrew, or Uncle Jr.; I'd ask running-related questions or geek out about gear. I'd research things to do in the next city I was conquering. It always worked. There was something about London that had me as stiff as a board. Gone was the thrill of anticipation I had felt for my previous races.

One of my favorite scenes in the film *Snatch* is, when the US gangster has to go see about his friend in the United Kingdom, he's clearly not happy about it. He turns to his bodyguard and says, "London . . . bad food, worse weather." I've never liked London. So when I booked my flight, I had bad feelings and planned on leaving the city immediately after the race.

I arrived at my Airbnb and wasn't sure why I was so down on the city. That April 2018, as is often true in the spring, the city's usual foggy and rainy weather had turned mostly cloud-free. Having won a lottery to gain my spot in the London race, I'd be competing in another Abbott World Marathon Majors run—this would complete number five of six. And after crushing fifteen marathons in just as many months, death had never crossed my mind once.

For years, I had romanticized climbing Mount Everest. In 1996, one of its deadliest years, twelve people died. Countless memoirs and survivors' accounts recounted gripping tales of falls, overzealous mountaineers, and amputees who still deal with survivors' guilt. The avalanches of 2014 and 2015 wiped out entire groups of would-be summiteers. And if that isn't terrible, I couldn't imagine the slow and painful death due to high-altitude cerebral edema and the mind-altering state of knowing you're dying, but with no Walgreens for pain pills, Harvard Medical School-trained doctor, or even God to scoop you up and help you out. If that doesn't get you, how about the sixty grand and two months' leisure time it takes just to risk it all? Summiting Everest makes marathoning sound like a Sunday stroll through Central Park.

However, people do die from attempting this 26.2-mile battle royale, as the race's origin shows. Twenty-one-year-old Francisco Lazaro died from electrolyte imbalance during the 1912 Olympic Marathon. In the 1980s and 1990s, lives were claimed in the New York City, Chicago, Marine Corps, and Boston races—four marathons I had just completed. Conditions range from heart attacks, body temperatures in the triple digits, and brain aneurysms to terrorist bombings. When most people think of marathons, they think of thick veins and a slow-resting heart rate; shapely calves; lean, long, fit bodies; all the energy required; and the joys of carb-loading.

For all the wondrous health benefits of marathoning, there are serious, undeniable dangers as well. Runners die—not at the rate of mountain climbers or BASE jumpers, but of strokes, heart attacks, and sepsis. In April 2018, Matt Campbell, who had competed on *MasterChef: The Professionals*, passed away at the London Marathon where I was competing, collapsing less than 10K from the finish line.

Significant research says that runners may be affected by muscle damage, torn knee ligaments, and kidney damage; these conditions can be isolated or chronic or both. These are real issues, ones that can cost people their lives out on the course. A heart attack, the silent killer that it is, may not look as gruesome as a tumble down Everest, but on the ground and writhing, runners too have known the pain of a physical barrier encountered—and the collapse that follows. Marathoning is, for that reason, a flawed way to stay in shape.

Campbell was younger and faster than I, so he had already been rushed to the hospital around the time darkness started to come upon me. It was hot. But I had just run Miami, which had had the red banner out signaling the dangers of the heat. The sun had blazed. But I had only left Hotlanta a few weeks ago, completing my second marathon in a row with temperatures soaring over eighty. But this was different. The BBC would officially mark this as the hottest marathon in the London event's history. Missing was their portent lecture of the real dangers to come.

For the first time, the sultry heat scared me. It scared the rest of the runners. The look in their eyes proclaimed not the typical angst of courageous soldiers but of battered warriors. The spectators meowed, the rays of the sunlight battering their voices like kittens being submerged in water. By mile ten, the mood didn't suddenly change; it was more like a dramatic intermission. We had no clue what was happening, but everyone knew the apocalypse was coming.

It wasn't until mile sixteen that I realized I was alone. There were no local friends, no Berlin crew, and Andrea wasn't on hand for only the second marathon out of all my races. In front of me was a man around fiftyish. His stride was smooth, and he was lean and tall. As I gained on him, not more than fifteen feet away, it happened: he checked his watch, clenched his chest, and dropped.

Melee ensued. Runners cared nothing of their times or personal records or what distance they were from the next water station. Ten people swarmed him like ants on spilled ice cream.

"Call the medics!" screamed one runner.

"We need a doctor!" screamed another.

I stopped. I wondered if there was anything I could do, but luckily, we were suddenly bombarded with a pack of trained physicians, and he was getting the care he needed.

I turned back to the race, and before I reached even another half mile, another male dropped a hundred feet in front of me. The scene was repeated another dozen times before I got to mile twenty. On the sidelines, I saw runners crying, sitting in their own vomit, and even more being tended to at every medical tent I passed. I imagined for a brief moment I was in the Marine Corps and this was what active duty looked like. Except there were no guns, bombers, or enemy lines—just 40,179 runners being pummeled by the electricity of solar energy.

I panicked. Sweat dripped from my nose. My body now felt the effects of fifteen months and hundreds of miles running; the blues turned into the reds. Music couldn't save me. I needed to listen for sirens, screams, and assure myself I could hear my own heartbeat. I looked around—there wasn't a familiar face in sight, my trackers were thousands of miles away, and no one gave me the nod. I was alone. And not the alone that one feels running your own race, but the alone one feels when every sound is censored around you in slow motion, yet moving toward the end. I had no clue what was going to happen to me. So, like always, I called my mother.

"Did you finish?" she asked, knowing that was when her phone normally rang on marathon Sunday.

"No, but I'm at mile twenty, and people are dropping like flies," I said. "I feel like I'm in a war zone."

My mom paused as if she was checking her notepad for the right words. "If you have to, walk away. You can always come back next year."

Next year? This was Abbott World Marathon Majors event number five. I was there for the gimcrack, that shiny, little medal that costs less than a dollar. I had gotten in this race through the lottery. Who knew when I'd be back or if I'd return?

According to David Goggins, we push ourselves and only reach 40 percent of our potential. In that moment, solar flares and UV rays be damned, the devil on one shoulder was telling me I was not being the best I could be. The angel on my other shoulder knew otherwise. I was committed to keeping my health intact. I listened to the angel that day.

Each person, Charles Moore included, must address the threshold of 40 percent perseverance for themselves. The fear of danger was not the excuse anymore. The wisdom of health, safety, and circumstance was my guiding context. Pushing myself was not just about me. My responsibility was to make it home to be with my wife and our soon-to-be-born child.

Thankfully, the high I had originally felt from marathoning suddenly returned. With three miles left, the dry, dull stiffness in my body became a loose, vibrant burst of energy. I stopped. I stretched. I kicked my knees up in the air to loosen my thighs. My hands interlocked, palms to the back of my head, and helped loosen and unstick my back. The tape on my ankles started to disconnect as my feet lunged on the curb to untighten my calves. The Ferrari engine started pumping blood all through my body. I was on an ultralight beam.

^^^

When I crossed the finish line, my mood was as dark as the weather. I pondered how I'd get back to my Airbnb. I could barely walk. My arms were too heavy to raise for a cab. My body was so riddled with holes from the sun's rays, it was hard to move in any direction. All I wanted to do was lay in the middle of the street and be carried to a bed. Any bed. Somehow, I made it back. Routinely, I'd immediately get in the shower, dress, relax no longer than fifteen minutes, and be off to dinner. That day was different. I went right to sleep. I did not pass go; I did not collect $200.

I woke up around midnight, London time—and I was starving. I hopped into the shower, dressed, and by 12:30 a.m., I was at a random restaurant that I have no explanation as to how I selected it. It was close by, it had steaks, and the first review (the only one I had read) seemed okay. The next day, I was off to change arenas for the rest of the week: Riga, Latvia, for the art nouveau architecture and Copenhagen, Denmark, to see the Henning Larsen-designed opera house. I loved the dichotomy of these two cultures. I couldn't wait for the six-month break I would have upon returning home.

Chapter 22

Hello Detroit!

The music bumped through the speakers of our Cadillac. To paraphrase Dorothy of *The Wizard of Oz* fame, "Lions and Tigers and Pistons, oh my!" Stevie was a part-time lover; Diana and Lionel's love was endless. Twelfth Street was no longer ablaze. And "Hello Detroit" was the song that woke me every morning.

Winter, spring, summer, and fall: the eighties in Detroit forged my formidable years. Back then, I went to Tigers games with my uncle Jr. and played touch football with my friends. Most of all, basketball was my favorite sport. In elementary and middle school, I played almost every day. And I was probably the only Jordan fan within 250 square miles; we were about 280 from Chicago. I had every pair of sneakers, every color wave. And when I went down to the camp in Atlanta for the AGLOA nationals tournament and ruined my entire outfit by playing basketball on the red soil, my parents didn't yell. They likened it to the eccentric nerdy kid who loved basketball, and we went shopping.

I never grew tall enough to consider basketball an option. In high school, at my uncle Jr.'s request, I tried out for the baseball team. "You're fast, you have great hand-eye coordination, and you know the game," he counseled.

All facts. If he had been a trial attorney, it would have been an open-and-shut case. But ladies and gentlemen of the jury, on day two of tryouts, as I was standing in the outfield, my friend Dwayne Burke ran up to me and said, "Go home, man. You look sick."

With a fighting bandit mentality, I ignored him. In the next inning, I swung the bat with the sluggish speed of a full-grown tree sloth. The coach yelled, "Moore, go home!"

Later that day, my mother, unaware of my ailment, assumed I didn't talk because I didn't make the team. Four hours later, she woke me and said, "You have chicken pox." And there went the Baseball Hall of Fame speech I'd been rehearsing.

Growing up in Detroit, we never needed a passport to cross into Canada. We traveled there often to throw dice, spin the roulette wheel, and yell, "Blackjack!" in the casinos that were not yet legal in the city. After prom, a group of us, Dwayne Burke included, decided we were going to cross the border and go to the casino. It was my idea, of course. I couldn't wait for the moment I'd waltz in with my dashing date; me draped in onyx pants, chalky jacket, and an ebony-black bow tie. "Moore . . . Charles Moore," I'd say the minute someone asked my name. It never happened. Turns out, the legal age to gamble was nineteen, and although we made it through the front door, we were all swiftly turned away.

I thought about that moment as I was walking up to the sign-in desk with the border police at the Detroit Free Press Marathon expo.

"Did you bring your passport?" Andrea asked.

I was such a pro at this point, I breezed through all the fine print for participants. "Of course not," I said, confident I didn't need it.

"Look," as she pointed to a bold statement about entry requirements.

You must have a valid passport to get your marathon packet, the sign read. Turns out that by mile three, we'd be crossing the Ambassador Bridge, prancing past the casinos before turning back to Detroit by way of the Detroit-Windsor Tunnel. I had never even looked at the course map or read the details. It just so happened that my passport was locked in my home safe, around six hundred miles away.

I had been in a situation similar before. On a trip to Naples, Italy, back in October 2009, Jayson, my banker buddy from college, had left his passport in Rome, not realizing you have to show it whenever you're staying in a hotel in Italy. I told him to get his roommate to snap a picture of his passport and send it to him. It worked. And ever since, I've kept a photo of my passport on my phone.

As per usual, my niece, Aria, and nephew Jaron accompanied me to the Detroit Institute of Arts Museum. It's a ritual whenever I return home to visit Detroit. I let nothing get in the way of our trip. Routinely, I make sure I find a few of the paintings that are for them. My cousin Deanna had visited the museum once. "Why would I go back? They have nothing there for us," she once told me. In a city that's 85 percent African American, the museum's

Black visitor rate is a jaw-dropping 5 percent.

I had no rebuttal for her at the time because she was absolutely right. But not unlike the marathon course, there are martyrs that bear the burden of assuring there are the proud and the few in the space. What I preached to the children of my siblings was, "Explore, be open, and stay optimistic." Like a favorite album on repeat, I sounded off. "Stand next to the Mickalene Thomas, Ari, I'd say to my niece" and "There goes your Ed Clark, Jaron, I'd point out to my nephew." We always ended with an exit through the gift shop to get them a token to remind them of our visit.

^^^

In all the previous out-of-town marathons, I'd scour the maps for the Marriott closest to the start or finish. Here in my hometown, I was staying only a short taxi ride away from the starting line at my mother's house. Early that Sunday morning, I bounced out of bed, got dressed, and raced downstairs to get my ride. As we were roaring down the Lodge Freeway, I was crushing a banana while confirming the starting line. I had no clue where the barricades would be or the setup. I arrived downtown only to find out we were blocked around three miles away from the start, and the driver had no clue how to get there. With only twenty minutes to go, I took a few deep breaths before I had a meltdown. And then I spotted a Bird electric scooter.

For grad school, I had been commuting weekly to Cambridge, Massachusetts, from New York City for about a year at this point and had spent the entire summer there. All summer, I'd been risking my life, cruising around Cambridge, hitting hills like I had safety gear on (I did not), riding a Bird scooter. Most cities thought they were a nuisance just because people drove them in the middle of the street and often left them wherever they pleased. But *I* knew differently, and this was an emergency. I didn't have my pilot's license and couldn't fly to the starting line . . . so a Bird was the next best thing. This little motorized hoverboard of sorts helped me blaze through the empty streets, dodge spectators, hop curbs, bypass barricades, and dash to the starting line on time.

When I finally arrived, I felt relieved and accomplished, almost like I'd already finished the race. As the gun went off, I came out cool. I felt more nervous about it being my hometown than anything. The head trash normally didn't start until at least mile sixteen, but here, it started by mile one. *Why am I here? What if I DNF in Detroit? What if I run into an old friend and they see me struggling?* Oddly enough, it was the first time I didn't tell myself it was the last marathon I was running. I knew it wasn't. I was here to make sure my presence in the room was felt. I was here to be friend, cousin, brother, or Uncle Jr. that someone could turn to and say, *He did that.*

The brisk, cold air that blew off the river chilled my body. I hoarded my energy in case I had to run . . . uh, turns out I did. I was running a marathon. My slower-than-usual pace was wreaking havoc on me. I felt cramps coming way too early, and my jacket wasn't really doing its job.

Because this race crossed into Canada, it was considered an international event, which comes with all sorts of threats of terrorism. There were specific rules in place for Detroit that were not to be broken. First, anyone not running was not allowed on the course. This was a typical rule, but often broken when a spectator's pony came prancing by and they wanted to give it a hug. Second, all runners must show their bibs at all times.

Another typical rule, but in this case, security personnel was on hand to address this whenever needed.

When we had gotten to Canada, I had thought about prom night all those years ago and being turned away. I thought about all the other trips I would make later with friends, losing wads of cash. (Never more than $200.) It was nice. Windsor was clean and healthy-looking. I almost felt like stopping for lunch; maybe a nice mound of poutine or a pile of Montreal smoked meat. I really just wanted to warm up in a greasy spoon diner because my fingers and toes were numb. Inside the tunnel back to the United States, I stopped for the proverbial selfie in front of the sign that signals the Canada/US border. When I got back to Detroit, I knew I needed to heat up and get moving.

My engine started revving up around mile twelve. My stride was unbroken while racing up Bagley Street. I saw two Black police officers on the curb to my left, and one motioned for me to unzip my jacket.

I'm freezing, I thought as I reluctantly followed orders. This Ferrari's engine was just taking off, so compliance didn't seem like too big a deal.

As I passed him, a White officer was just behind him. He jumped off his post in front of me and placed his left arm out as his right hand went for his pistol.

Is this guy seriously going for his gun?

"I need to see your bib!" he shouted.

"You can say it, but don't you dare put your hands on me, or by the time I'm done suing you, I'll be renting your home out for extra income," I blurted out as I came to a standstill.

No sooner did the words leave my mouth than two White male runners stood by my side. One whipped out his phone and started recording. The other yelled for the Black officers just feet behind us. "Touch him, and I'll be sure this recording is delivered to the Free Press," the first guy said.

"His bib is clearly showing," one of the Black officers said.

While the officer was holstering his weapon, the lyrics "You're a fighter, you're a lover/You're strong and you recover..." danced in my head. I just wanted to run my race. These two men—or should I say comrades—ran with me for the next two miles. Their anger and instant reactions reminded me of all the men and women who chose love over hate. The people who were willing to stand up for what's right and not sit back in silence. They were fighters.

In fact, one told me he was a black belt and was willing to take that guy down. I'm glad he didn't. I'd rather be in the paper for challenging the status quo of what a marathoner looks like instead of becoming Swiss cheese after my bodyguards tried to take out a cop.

^^^

It was freezing. In the last three races, I couldn't wait to find respite in an air-conditioned room. Now I begged for warmth. The chills that ran down my spine reminded me of those formidable years I had spent waiting for a bus in freezing temperatures while growing up in Michigan. I couldn't wait to embrace my family and get back to my mother's house to change and go out to Buddy's Pizza for dinner.

Every time I'm in Detroit, it just feels like home. But running its marathon felt like we, the city and I, were giving each other a big hug after spending so many years together. Thanks for the memories, Detroit.

Chapter 23

Black Men Run Marathons.

The third time is a charm. I didn't know what to expect—maybe an entourage, bodyguards, and a band playing my theme song. Definitely some theme music because every good hero should have some. As I sped down the FDR Drive in November 2018, heading to the ferry, I was excited for a third go at the New York City Marathon. The weather was perfect—low fifties, no wind, and the humidity was even-tempered.

At the South Ferry station, I met again with Anca, who handled marathon starts much like I did: always take a taxi, the walk to the starting line is the best warmup, and never be on time. I think it's why we're still friends.

"We're early," she said.

"Yeah, just early enough to make the wave of runners behind us."

This ferry ride was different. We sat in silence. She, checking her phone and watch while eating a banana; me, thinking about what this race would be like.

One thing that crossed my mind as we approached the starting line was *who* was at the starting line. I was reminded of the NYRR's mission statement: Help and inspire through running. *Isn't that interesting?* I thought. Here we are, at another marathon starting line, and I'm thinking about their mission and diversity policy.

Diversity has become something of a buzzword. While this doesn't make it any less meaningful or relevant, it is important to clarify exactly what it entails. At the core of most diversity initiatives is a desire to represent people from all backgrounds within an organization or community. From colleges to media companies, many organizations are taking an active role in ensuring sufficient DEIA (diversity, equity, inclusion, and accessibility) measures. One way to elevate diversity is for the institution in question to home in on DEIA, creating a committee or initiative focused on this practice.

The idea is to include members of underrepresented groups, provide equitable access to training and leadership development opportunities, and ultimately boost employee satisfaction and retention. This was the case later when the NYRR would have a public debate over racism among its organization's employees. If you can't figure out how to promote a healthy, diverse environment in the office, how will that spill over into race participation? I'll answer that—it won't. And yet again, it showed when I arrived at the starting line. Again, there were hundreds and hundreds of people, and when I panned my camera to record the energy, I couldn't help but feel a bit of sorrow.

Diversity is perhaps the best-represented part of the DEIA umbrella. These characteristics include but are not limited to national origin, race, language, disability, ethnicity, gender expression, sexual orientation, gender identity, socioeconomic status, veteran status, and age. The term also includes differences among people based on their thought patterns and lived experiences. Specific standards should be set within organizations to keep on track, with regular follow-ups to monitor progress.

While diversity focuses on representation, equity is founded on the consistent and systematic, fair, and impartial treatment of all people no matter their background. The practice is designed to comprehensively advance equity, or equal and fair treatment, for all individuals—extending to people of color and others who have historically been marginalized, underserved, or adversely affected in the way of access to opportunity. In addition to Black people and others who identify as members of the BIPOC (Black, Indigenous, and people of color) community, this equity must extend to religious minorities; LGBTQ* (lesbian, gay, bisexual, transgender, and queer) people; those with disabilities; and additional groups negatively affected by poverty or inequality. Regarding how an organization might work toward greater equity, its policies and programming could nonetheless perpetuate systemic barriers to opportunities.

Inclusion is the recognition, appreciation, and use of everyone's talents and skills. The objective here is to incorporate the unique characteristics of people from all backgrounds in order to strengthen the organization in question. A well-established ideal set forth in the DEIA concept, inclusion moves beyond diversity by serving as not only a call for representation but as a call to action. This is largely rooted in organizational culture, as the entity in question must foster an environment of collaboration, fairness, and flexibility—connecting diverse people to the organization and leveraging diversity to make sure all members feel comfortable participating and contributing to the fullest extent. Like diversity, an organization's inclusion initiatives must be periodically assessed as a means of quality control.

Accessibility is the design, construction, development, and maintenance of programs, facilities, information and communication technologies, and services such that all individuals—including people with disabilities—can access them with ease. Equally, these same people must be able to completely and independently use these programs and systems.

While most organizations are well-meaning in their intent to promote DEIA, there are several pitfalls to diversity measures. In my experience running seventeen marathons so far, none of them had passed the eyeball test. Would today be different?

∧∧∧

Anca had been much more consistent at training than I. And it showed. I felt sluggish for the first few miles, as if my shoes had been weighed down by cement. My emotions, contemplating all the issues that plagued marathoning, were weighing on me. After she shot out like a cannon, we had to part ways before we hit the third mile. I slowed to a walk.

At this point, we were still packed like a swarm of bees. I've lived in New York City since 2005 and had run this race twice already. But I still hadn't gotten used to the curves and angles that make up unfamiliar boroughs like Staten Island and the southern neighborhoods of Brooklyn. I felt like a tourist again: crossing the Verrazzano-Narrows Bridge, trucking through Bay Ridge, and gliding up Fourth Avenue.

I hadn't expected to see Andrea much, if at all, this time. She was eight months pregnant by now and carrying around an entire second person. By mile four, I called her to check in.

"How are you feeling?" she answered, her voice brighter than my mood.

"I'm fresh out of juice, and I'm still in Brooklyn." I didn't want to alarm her, but I felt terrible.

I could hear the ruffling of papers in the background. "I'm checking your pace, and it seems to be good," she said, trying to jostle the doubt and malaise out of me.

"The pace is one thing, but my feet are telling me to walk into this café and order myself a cappuccino."

The silence on the other end reminded me of how bad my jokes were. Or maybe she knew I was fishing for more words of encouragement. "You got this," she said. "This is only what, your eighteenth marathon?"

The next few miles felt lonely. Strange, because this stretch of Fourth Avenue boasts a nonstop crowd of civilians—screaming, cheering, and handing out homemade energy treats. Once we got near the Barclays Center, I saw the Black Men Run group. It felt differently this time. I hadn't noticed them in the prior two races there. But I hadn't been thinking about diversity, equity, inclusion, and accessibility back then.

This begs the question: How can these spaces incorporate and elevate DEIA initiatives with minimal bias and without being self-serving? How might race organizers use the acronym not as a buzzword, but as something actionable; an active measure to include, accommodate, and represent those who have long been underserved? These are key considerations for those looking to embrace or simply understand DEIA.

I blocked the idea. I had to table it for another time. It was affecting my race and eating away at my energy. One marathon at a time, Charles. Mile twenty-five of the New York City Marathon, mile one of the DEIA. Thankfully, I didn't have much longer to go in my adopted hometown.

After the race, I got a text from Andrew: *Check this out, bro.* He sent me a picture of his medal.

Wait, you're in NYC? I had no clue he was there running today. *Let's meet up tomorrow,* I responded.

We met at Balthazar, one of my favorite restaurants downtown in SoHo. It would be the first time we had actually sat down and talked. It was at that breakfast I learned that Andrew not only runs marathons, but he's an art collector as well. It's incredible how much in common you'll find if you just talk to people.

Chapter 24

Swag Surfin'

Every eye is on you, and out of the corner of your eye, the gold glistens, signaling to all who look upon you that you have won—that you have done something, achieved some level of glory worth celebrating and commemorating. Whether it's the Vince Lombardi Trophy or a high school letterman jacket, that sparkle seems to leap into the air, exuding an aura of greatness along with it. It is the flame of victory and persistence, one that no one needs to light and that everyone must respect.

Call it an award. Call it a piece of memorabilia. Trophies, medals, ribbons: they are just trinkets unless we understand the significance the holder ascribes to them. Ask the person who won it or the person wearing it or hoisting it into the air what the accomplishment means. Ask them, by extension, what all their hard work and effort have meant.

No one in the NBA ever showed up to claim a championship ring from the finals without first training for a lifetime and certainly not without first competing against the best players in the world. Every college athlete knows—and most of them learned when they were still in elementary school—that the award isn't made of metal but rather the sweat they left behind.

Nonathletes get it too. Whenever you see a wedding ring, that signifies an accomplishment as well. Two people have, despite the odds stacked against them, found each other, agreed to look out for each other, and then go marching off to a life very different from the only life they've known. It's worth a trophy.

Your high school diploma, a certificate of appreciation, even the scorecard from your last round of golf: each one is a symbol of a goal realized and pursued—of a life lived and lived successfully. You get the win, you take the trinket, and although you go on your way, the accomplishment departs along with you because of the object used to symbolize it.

So when I walked up to the starting line to run my nineteenth marathon, I knew why I was there and what I was going for. Why? My wife, now the mother of my son, would be running around New York City with *Il Principe* Charles II. What I didn't know then was how energetic he would be. An athlete in the making. He runs, he jumps, he climbs. Do they make ironman races for kids?

^^^

Only months prior, I would walk across the stage at Harvard University: twice. Once to get my diploma—a masters in museum studies—the second time, to be presented the Titus & Venus Legacy Award at Harvard's Black Graduation Ceremony.

I remember being told about the ceremony in 2018, which, even as a Black person, I didn't initially understand. "You must go to this," Sylvia, a friend of mine who graduated a year before me said. "It's the only place during graduation we get to celebrate *us* the way we do it. It's basically the BBQ."

I was sold.

In early April 2019, I was informed via email that I had won the Titus & Venus Legacy Award. At the time, I had no clue who they were or if they were real people. What I did know is the award was given to a graduating student who had displayed dedication to improving the Black community through their academic and/or community service during their time at Harvard. I never questioned my dedication to uplifting the people and the conversations about us as Black people. But I still pondered the need for separation. Why do we need our own ceremony at Harvard? I learned that it wasn't that we weren't accepted at the main ceremony; we just weren't equally represented or celebrated.

In 2016, a *Harvard Gazette* staff writer named Christina Pazzanese wrote a piece titled "To Titus, Venus, Bilhah, and Juba." She confirmed my worst fears, stating, "Aiming to confront present-day vestiges of long-ago slavery at the University, Harvard officials today celebrated some of the people whose lives and toil remained invisible for so long, dedicating a plaque to four colonial-era slaves." I felt conflicted.

On the day of the ceremony, one of the organizers, Princess, found me and ushered me to the back room. There was a churning in the bottom of my stomach. It felt like I had eaten something highly fibrous and it wanted to come out. "You're to come to the back for the meet and greet," she said.

My stomach settled a bit, but the intensity was heightened when I saw so many important people laughing and carrying on as if they had all heard the punchline to a joke that was about me. There was Dean Bridget Terry Long and Congresswomen Ayanna Pressley and Jahana Hayes. There was John Silvanus Wilson, ex-president of Morehouse College and newly appointed senior adviser and strategist to the university's president.

I had no clue what was going on, why I was there, and if I'd find a bucket to fill with all my accumulated sweat. My nerves calmed as Dr. Cornel West entered. It was like a bottle full of lightning had been released as he strode into the room. In his presence, one finds that they spend their time trying to catch said lightning, only to find themselves exhausted, the lightning finding its way back into the bottle once he leaves. I tapped my superpowers, and once my swag surfin' was done, I gathered my crew and went to dinner.

^^^

My nineteenth and final marathon felt like a victory lap. I jogged, I waved, and I blotted. The run was so smooth that the entire time felt like it was a Groundhog Day of one-milers. I took in the spectators like they were all there just for me, and I appreciated them. The sweat trickled down my face, but the wind caught it before it could get to my eyebrows. I was in a groove.

At the time, I didn't know it would be my last race. When I had learned about the Abbott World Marathon Majors early in 2017, I knew it was something I wanted to accomplish. I ran New York City, then Boston, then Berlin, then Chicago before closing in on London. I only had Tokyo to go. After some homework, giving Google Translate a hefty workout, I was going to have to overcome a huge hurdle to get into Tokyo. I signed up for a charity spot in the 2019 race, casually raising the $3,000 required to get in, only to find out they take just the first five thousand runners who reach the goal. In the Facebook group, Tokyo Marathon, I was told everyone signs up the first day, pays the donation, then raises the money. I felt like Holofernes of Apocrypha fame, and my head had just gotten chopped off. So by the time the news came out regarding the 2020 Tokyo race, I was on it. I signed up, dropped the three grand, and knew I'd cross the fundraising bridge at a later date.

^^^

In the summer of 2019, I decided to start another marathon: a doctorate. Most of the summer was spent studying for the Graduate Record Examinations (GREs) and deciding which programs I'd be applying to. I applied to Columbia, Berkeley, Brown, Harvard, Princeton, and Yale. The process was grueling. There were the GREs, researching the departments and professors, applications, and the dreaded essays. Overall, the essays were straightforward: tell us about your life, the academic work you want to do, and the professors and resources at our university that will help you accomplish your research goals. One university, after clicking the box that I identified as Black or African American, triggered an additional short essay about what diversity meant to me. Wait. *I have to write an additional essay on this?* I thought.

I was shocked. I had no words. I pondered the idea for weeks. Then I thought about the similarities among this question, academia, art museums, and endurance running—specifically marathoning. So I wrote an essay titled "Black People Don't Run Marathons," which read:

Black people don't run marathons. In 2016, as I approached the New York City Marathon starting point on the Verrazzano-Narrows Bridge in Staten Island, I looked around at all the excited—soon-to-be accomplished—faces. There were very few Black ones. Diversity is seeing one's own identity affirmed and celebrated at every turn. That day, I finished the marathon and went on to complete eighteen more over the next three years. Along the way, I encouraged and inspired six of my friends, all African American, to complete their first marathon. To continue to be an example to others, I ran the 26.2-mile race in Rome, Boston, Chicago, Berlin, London, and other cities to show my friends the possibilities.

When I ran the Rome marathon, I wasn't surprised to be possibly the only African American in the race. However, running in cities like Atlanta, Miami, Birmingham, and Washington, DC, I felt a glaring lack of representation. "Black people don't run marathons," wrote Marcus Ryder, published in *The Guardian*, "because they don't see people like them at running clubs where they train." At every turn, if I saw a Black person, they almost always gave me "the nod." You know that slight tilt of the head that says to the other Black person you recognize their presence. According to a survey of 12,000 runners taken by *Running USA* in 2011, 90 percent of marathoners were White, while 1.6 percent were Black. It is clear that even elitist athletic activities are unfortunately not dissimilar to art museums: they historically and presently lack diversity. As a result, I plan to use my experiences and bring visibility to opportunities to change these narratives.

If we abandon all hope, ye who enter here, we abandon all dreams. At my core, I've always been a dreamer. As an adolescent, I dreamed about living in Italy, ordering wines and champagnes in Italian, and cruising the ruins and squares of ancient cities. As a teenager, I dreamed of moving to New York City, working on Wall Street, and dining in fine restaurants in my well-tailored suit. In college, I regretted never applying to Harvard; I knew I had the chops to get in. As an adult, I wanted to see operas all over the world, learn to play the oboe, and rear caterpillars to butterflies. Now I dream of someday being called Dr. Charles Moore.

What happens if you abandon all hope? Dreams deferred will *stink like rotten meat.*

Back to that groove I was in. I finished that race. My nineteenth marathon in record time. It wasn't my personal record, but a record of my person. I have no memories of the actual race. It was a blur. What I do recall is the moment I arrived at mile twenty-six, with two-tenths of a mile to go, I stopped. I looked at my watch, checked my phone, and took in the moment. I wasn't dreaming. It was very real. And as I crossed the finish line and was awarded my medal, I posed for a picture. I was at the final stage of a peak of performance: a dream realized.

Chapter 25

Ahmaud the Brave!

When I heard about the circumstances surrounding Ahmaud Arbery's murder in 2020, it sounded all too familiar. Here was a man who had been getting his regular exercise, working out for the rush of it to keep himself in shape so he might live a little healthier and a little longer, and he was cut down by a lynch mob like so many before him. It is important to recount his story here so that the enormity of the transgression is clear.

Ahmaud was on the side of a residential road, a little less than three hundred miles west of where my uncle Jr. lives in Georgia. He was in one lane, and the Ford F-150, the one carrying his killers, was in the other. One of those killers was standing up in the back of the truck as if watching for prey—watching for an innocent life to steal.

When Ahmaud and the F-150 crossed paths, the murderers accosted him. The three men shouted at him—and what did he hear? Not the cheers that I had garnered while running any of my nineteen marathons. Their words were not of encouragement, not even of questioning, but of accusation. He had dared to run that day. The sweat on his back and the air in his lungs were evidence of what had offended that band in the F-150. He had dared to venture outside and live his life, to sprint and jog around the Georgia land that was his home.

That was all it took: To live, to breathe, to be; it was enough for those three hateful ghouls to take chase. One run turned into another. Intending to exercise, Ahmaud instead found himself running for his life. It pains me to do so, but I have imagined the feeling he must have gotten in his stomach, the anxious cramp that must have swelled inside him when instead of running for pleasure, he was running to survive.

Ahmaud put up a noble fight. He and one of his murderers grappled over the shotgun that the three of them had aimed at him. The odds were too much, though. Surely, this decorated athlete would have made short work of any of his attackers, but they were three against his one. They had gone out marauding for souls and found one in Ahmaud Arbery.

Ahmaud: a runner, just like me. Just like my uncle Jr. Just like many other Black people who sprint, jog, or run marathons. Ahmaud, whose death would become like a bell, tolling away the minutes of the hate that was clearly still festering in Georgia, just miles away from where my uncle Jr. runs daily.

Uncle Jr. later confessed to me that this incident caused him so much grief that he stopped running. I only ran outside on race day. But he had run outside almost daily for decades, just for the love of it.

When the jury found those killers guilty of malicious murder, it was a sign that the truth could prevail. However, that something like this could happen in the first place was also a sign. Every run Ahmaud had gone on, he had taken his life into his own hands. He had risked it all for that runner's high, even if there was no way for him to know for certain he would survive. In America, it turns out, there is more at risk in preparing for a race than a torn ligament or a sprained ankle. If you happen to be a Black runner, it can become a combat sport when it never should have been that and should never be that again.

For the moment, I'm just thankful that, once again, guys like Uncle Jr. began to run this season, hoping that what happened to Ahmaud Aubrey will never happen again.

^^^

In 2013, *The Guardian* published Ryder's article "Why don't black people run marathons?" It examined a phenomenon to which many people in the United States would attest, at least anecdotally: at marathons nationwide, Black people make up only a small portion of all the runners.

The piece reads, in part:

While the gender barrier seems to be tumbling, there seems to be another when it comes to distance racing: black people do not run marathons.

This is all the more surprising considering that nearly all the top marathon runners, both male and female, are African. The one statistic I have found, from *Running USA*'s biannual National Runner Survey, reveals that only 1.6% of marathon runners in America are African-American, compared with 90% Caucasian, 5.1% Hispanic, and 3.9% Asian/Pacific Islander.

It is, however, both dismissive and incorrect to say that Black people are not running marathons. Whether or not Ryder meant to be hyperbolic, the reality is that many runners, because they do not see Black people participating in marathons, may take it literally. There is value in analyzing the current statistics that are emblematic of the exclusion and discrimination that have at times loomed large over the sport, but they gloss over important exceptions. If we simply say, "Black people don't run marathons," we are casting aside the rich, decades-long history that Black pioneers have written—and the significance behind their willingness to enter a space where few others looked like them or shared their cultural experiences.

Take Ted Corbitt, for example. He was the founding president of NYRR, New York City's premier running group and one of the largest athletic organizations in the world. Born in 1919, he became a luminary in the marathon during an era when the participants were even more homogeneous than today. Corbitt would run more than twenty miles every day between Broadway and the Harlem River, from the Bronx to Manhattan. In his son Gary's own words, though, "My father always told me that he wasn't alone—that there were other great Black American distance runners. I didn't know just how rich the history was until I started to look into it myself."

The younger Corbitt, for his part, has committed himself to preserving the often-overlooked history of Black distance running. He has traced the beginnings of the sport within the Black community to its start as a whole in the United States. Going all the way back to the late nineteenth century, we find Frank Hart, a Black immigrant who was born Fred Hichborn in 1858. When he arrived in the United States in the 1870s, Hart participated in what was then the country's top sport: marching. Marchers, over multiday events, would run and walk between checkpoints. These races spanned hundreds of miles, predating the modern ultramarathon. Hart, who worked full time at a Boston grocery store, was one of the first athletes to go professional as a marcher—and preceded founders of the running movement in America.

Approximately a century after Hart was dominating marching, Marilyn Bevans ran a marathon with a finishing time of 3:04:32, winning the George Washington's Birthday Marathon in Beltsville, Maryland. Bevans was the first African American woman to win a US marathon, and soon after, she stacked her résumé further, finishing fourth at the Boston Marathon with a time of 2:55:52. In 1977, she became the first African American to medal at the Boston Marathon, beating her original time with a second-place finish at 2:51:12. It was the era of Nike, the ascent of distance running to cultural extravaganza, and a shining moment for Black excellence in a sport that less than forty years later, a *Guardian* headline would claim had no Black participants at all.

Bevans has since said of her experience, "I enjoyed training. I loved training. I wasn't thinking about being the first [Black woman], honestly. I just wanted to be the best and compete. I wanted to win, and I knew with hard work I was going to have a shot."

Tony Reed, like Bevans, has also cemented his name in the annals of Black distance running: Not only was he the first Black person to finish a marathon on all seven continents, but he has run marathons in all US states. In total, Reed has finished 131 marathons. His contributions in opening up the sport to more Black people than ever before are undeniable and result in large part from him shining a light on all of the Black men and women who have helped build distance running into the sport that it is.

Reminiscing about the 2004 Saint Louis Marathon, Reed said in an interview with *Runner's World*, "The kids who were watching the race started running along with me, and I was talking with them. That's when it really hit me. For these Black kids to see a Black runner in a race, I was kind of like a role model, and I never thought about myself being a potential role model for people who see me when I'm out there running." It is this line of thinking that has kept Reed motivated to do the important outreach work that he does and to reveal the truth about Black people and marathons as opposed to the anecdotal misconceptions that have persisted.

Black Americans have contributed to the growth of long-distance running in other ways without launching a nonprofit or winning a medal. Tiffany Chenault, a sociology professor at Salem State University, has said of her running experience, "Running is really a microcosm of a larger society. So even though it should be all welcoming and inclusive, it's not." Chenault has since pivoted her academic research to focus on racial, social, and economic factors that may prevent Black athletes from running as a hobby.

Global distance running has become, we should note, a showcase of the latest talent to emerge from specific regions of Kenya, Ethiopia, and Eritrea. The world has watched in awe as generational talents Eliud Kipchoge, Mo Farah, Haile Gebrselassie, and Kenenisa Bekele have exhibited just what is possible from the human body. Their conditioning and achievements are landmarks in the modern science of sports medicine.

Black Americans have also reached the pinnacle of distance running in recent years. Keflezighi was thirty-nine years old in 2014 when he placed first at the Boston Marathon. He was the most recent American to win the event, and no other American has ever won Boston, New York, and an Olympic medal. After retiring, he parlayed his fame as America's fastest marathoner into a career in media and philanthropy, running for NYRR Team for Kids, among other charities.

There are many other lesser-known Black runners whose journeys and accomplishments have been no less impressive than Keflezighi's. Aliphine Tuliamuk came in first at the US Olympic Trials for the marathon in 2020. She then went on to represent the United States at the Tokyo Olympics in 2021, competing at the highest level while she was also breastfeeding her newborn baby. Although on a much smaller stage than Tuliamuk, Nathan Martin, a thirty-one-year-old who has been running since childhood, broke the marathon speed record for Black American men in Chandler, Arizona, in 2021.

Asked about his beginnings in the sport, he revealed how important having supporters can be: "I was pretty hesitant at first, but by eighth grade, [my teachers] convinced me."

Martin's story is the story of Black distance runners in the United States: of course, Black people run, and if we continue to address inequalities in the sport, tackle safety concerns outdoors, and encourage young Black people to get started sooner rather than later, then the statistics will bear that out. Organizations such as Black Men Run, the Civil Rights Race Series, Black Girls RUN!, GirlTrek, and the NBMA are all doing the tough and critical work changing the narrative around Black people and running, breaking myths, and celebrating heritage.

As we bring to light false notions, they will stop perpetuating themselves. The truth is that Black people do run and have always run—even before the sport had fully taken shape. By facilitating the development of a more equitable sport and hobby, a more diverse population can discover the pain of miles eight, twelve, and twenty—as well as the incomparable joy of reaching mile twenty-six and the finish line that follows—but more importantly, the health benefits of consistent running.

Speaking of Black people running...I had a lot more running to do myself. I hadn't run a marathon or even prepared for one since Ahmaud Arbery's tragic murder, and I needed to blow off a little (maybe a lot of) steam. I wasn't necessarily committed to dedicating my next marathon to Ahmaud, but he would certainly be in my thoughts as I competed. That couldn't be helped. And I still had one more Abbott World Marathon Majors event left to go—Tokyo. I had planned it out for some time; Tokyo was going to take place in March 2020. And nothing, absolutely nothing, was going to get in my way.

Chapter 26

Ground Zero.

I couldn't have been more thrilled to complete my long-standing goal to run in all six Abbott World Marathon Majors. I had my plane ticket to Tokyo, Japan, booked. And my hotel spot near the finish line was secured. All I needed to do was stay in relatively fair shape and not get injured. Even in my midforties, I felt I could manage that.

By mid-February, I started to get phone calls from some concerned family members and well-wishers.

"I'm sorry to tell you," Matt said. "Cancel your trip to Japan, bro."

"I'm hearing we're at the start of the plague," DJ told me.

"I *will* be running the Tokyo Marathon," I insisted to both of them.

And when the email came in the beginning of February reading <*Attention!* ► *Important Announcement for Tokyo Marathon 2020 Participants*, I admit I got a little nervous. But still, I opened the email immediately and found bib pickup times, the pickup location, and the confirmation of my bib number.

But as the crescendo of dramatic music continued through the week, signifying what was coming in the world, I knew I'd be calling the airline for a flight credit and canceling my hotel.

The next email had the subject line *IMPORTANT INFORMATION RELATED TO TOKYO MARATHON 2020*. I felt a cramp in my stomach that slowed my hand movement as I opened the email.

*On February 17, we announced the final decision for the 2020 event through our official website . . . *Please be advised that all registered runners for 2020 will have a guaranteed entry to the 2021 event.*

Tokyo was postponed till 2021?!

I was crushed. I didn't cry, but I wish I had. My disappointment couldn't be wiped away from my face. Every day, I had thought about how I would feel when I would finally sail across the finish line. Who would award me with my six-star medal? What champagne would I open to celebrate? And how none of that mattered at all. If I had done absolutely nothing, that would've been great too. If I lost something I had worked hard for, I wouldn't have been happy, but I still would have been proud of myself for putting maximum effort into preparation and execution of the task. But being ready and not being able to compete almost felt worse than if I had gone to Tokyo and not finished the race for any reason. I don't fear failure. I fear not trying.

As we know now, the global pandemic didn't just end there. So by the fall of 2020, I felt numb. I hadn't run a single mile all year. I ate like a king thanks to the Royal 35 Steakhouse next door. They sold me and a few neighbors dry-aged American

Wagyu steaks out the front door at cost weekly. And every week, my body stiffened from the lack of movement. If I walked fifteen hundred steps in a day, it was a good day. Mentally, I was shattered. I needed this pandemic to be over so I could get my spirits back up and hopefully get back to moving.

By December 2020, I already expected another email and barely got up the nerve to open it once I finally received it.

1) Which Event to Defer

Please choose to defer your entry to either the "Tokyo Marathon 2021" or the "Tokyo Marathon 2022."

-Tokyo Marathon 2021 Sunday, October 17, 2021 (provisional)

-Tokyo Marathon 2022 Sunday, March 6, 2022 (provisional)

It was brutal. Of course, I selected October 17, 2021, which would eventually be canceled. And once again, March 6, 2022 . . . canceled.

By this time, I was moving a little bit more, but I still hadn't run a single mile. I felt like a star athlete who had been forced into retirement—albeit prematurely. But I vividly recall, right after a three-peat of championships, Jordan had announced his retirement. He would come back almost two years later, just to double down and three-peat a second time.

In April 2022, I started running again. If marathon running had jerseys like in basketball, I would have chosen to wear number 45. My Jordan-esque comeback started as I signed up for the 2022 New York City Marathon, a race I would run for the fifth time. I had packed on an extra twenty pounds thanks to good eating and virtually no movement, but mentally, it was like I was at ground zero. I had forgotten how to train, and I had to regain my grit.

I changed shoes for the first time in ages. I decided on the Nike Air Zoom Alphafly NEXT%s. The shoes that were once banned for elite distance runners and in the Olympics, citing "technology doping." Hey, I was coming back from a hiatus at forty-five years old; I'd take all the advantages I could get. You feel like a kangaroo when you put these sneakers on, they've got so much bounce.

It would be the first time I'd set an actual schedule, and I even trained outdoors. I ran three to four times per week, averaging six to ten miles per run. I returned to a healthier diet and started to shed the weight. If you eat healthy and keep active, you'll maintain a healthy body weight. It's funny how that works. But as the weight dropped off, my confidence level went the other way. I felt like . . . like I could run an *ultra*marathon!

"Are you crazy?" Andrea replied when I told her what I was thinking. "What is that, anyway?"

"An ultra is technically anything more than a marathon, but they typically start at 50K—basically thirty-one miles at a minimum."

As I was confirming my entry in the 2022 New York City Marathon, I was also seeking out where I could run a 50K—either before or after. Eventually, I landed on Dallas, Texas. I needed a new challenge and an ultramarathon just seemed to do the trick.

^^^

On race day, I at least knew I looked great. I had on an all-black Tracksmith T-shirt and all-black Tracksmith running tights with a gray stripe down the side. A ciele x Tracksmith black cap. And the equalizer: blue Nike Air Zoom Alphafly NEXT%s. I looked like I had just stepped off the cover of *Runner's World* magazine.

The gear felt like protective body armor because on the inside, I felt like a stand-up comic trying out new material in front of a rowdy crowd. *I've done this four times already,* I kept telling myself. As I boarded the ferry to Staten Island that morning, it felt like my first time. I checked out the people and observed their excitement. Of course, someone on that ferry hadn't done this ride before. Someone on that ferry wouldn't finish the race. Someone on that ferry would get their six-star medal at the end. Someone on that ferry would be running their twentieth marathon. Wait. This was my fifth time running this event, but it would be my twentieth time running 26.2 miles in a day. By the time I got up to the starting line, I'd forgotten about the protective cool apparel I was wearing. All I thought about was crossing the starting line and then the finish line.

This would end up being the easiest marathon I'd run— physically and mentally. I ripped through the crowd of runners like I was the only one there. I sprinted past mile markers like the wind behind me pushed away all doubt. The entire race was a blur. It seemed to climax only when I got home to shower. I was ready for a steak. But this time, I'd earned it. Next stop: Dallas.

Chapter 27

Ripping through.

Running in a large group, you look around at the faces, and it's easy for moments or even minutes at a time to lose track of the road underneath your feet and the scenes passing by you on either side. You see only the faces, huffing and puffing just like yours, glancing around stealthily at all the other faces too. While you pump your arms into the thick wind and your toes tap lightly against the pavement, your mind is ambling along most refreshingly. You can *think*, and with every passing mile, you get to think a little more.

The running community captivated me as quickly as it did much for this reason. I felt whenever I lined up for another marathon that I was a part of something—that all these new friends and I were angling for the same spectacular feeling, the same sense that we understood ourselves better than we had when we had woken up that morning. This community transcends geography, and it transcends interests: you may meet a few dozen runners during a race and never find a single person who thinks like you do, except that you're both passionate about running.

That passion is *enough*.

With that kind of passion around you, with that sort of collective effort, you do not need to look hard to come up with some motivation for yourself. It's inspiring enough to see all those people running alongside you. Even though your time is your own and you know that only you can run your race for yourself, you still share all the oxygen around you. You are still running on the same road, whether you finish first or last. The community of runners, as manifested any time there is a 5K, a 10K, a half-marathon, a marathon, or *something more*.

I am going to talk about that *something more*, the edge to which I often wandered up to and which I only crossed over after deep reflection and a whole lot of training. It took inspiration too, of course. The great challenges always do, in order to achieve something that you have never achieved before, particularly something that *seems* on the cusp of impossible. That *something more* requires you to look inside yourself and embrace all of the nuances, to know yourself as you couldn't know yourself at the breakneck, never-look-around speed at which you live your life.

Before I tell you about my recent challenge, let me tell you about my friend, Oliver Ventura. A second-generation Dominican, Oliver has been a close friend of mine since we were undergrads at Michigan State University. Oliver and I get along naturally. We understand each other, which makes it easy for us to talk openly and to say what is really on our minds. As well, we look out for each other. We talk about what is going in our lives and what our goals are.

After finishing college, I moved to New York City and Oliver moved to Nashville. He wound up in Austin sometime later.

When I started running marathons in 2016, he seemed interested in joining me. Fitness had never been a part of our friendship, though. Oliver's parents had never lived a healthy lifestyle, which meant that he had inherited some of their unhealthy habits. All his life, he has struggled with being slightly overweight.

As I was racking up medals, swag, memorabilia, and trinkets from all the races that I was running, Oliver picked up the sport too. He would report back to me, telling me about the jog he had gone for the evening before. The distances were short, but he was doing it. He saw how much running had come to mean to me, and he had claimed it as his own as well.

So what was the *problem*?

The problem was that Oliver never signed up for a race. I explained to him what the races meant to me, how I felt like I was a part of something, how they motivated me to keep setting my goals higher. For years, I *longed* to get that text: *I signed up!* or *My first race is next month!* or *Look what I'm doing!*

We talked it out, and Oliver agreed to a 5K right in Dallas. The plan was to run that Saturday, but when Oliver arrived, I realized that he had neither signed up for the race nor packed his shoes, only days before race day he'd tell me. No matter: he was there with me in Texas, and we would make it happen. I didn't have to long for any text. Rather, I could take it upon myself to inspire my friend. I put on my best Al Pacino and did a spot-on re-creation of the *Any Given Sunday* speech. It worked, and since I had already paid for his entry by then, there was nothing standing between him and his first finish.

That was the first race I had ever experienced from the sidelines. I wanted him to have his moment while I supported him through this journey. Besides, I'd be running an ultramarathon the next day. I watched one of my oldest, closest friends barrel through decades of naysaying and a lifetime of questioning. *Can I be healthy? Will this work for me?*

Oliver crushed that 5K. When I met him at the finish line, I reminisced about all the times that he had told me how inspiring I was to him. I felt a chill as I told him that today, *he* was the one inspiring me. He had met his deepest fears and stared them down. His challenge had persisted, and he had persisted along with it. That day, Oliver was the most courageous runner I knew.

In the aftermath of Oliver's first 5K, I had to rethink all of my perspectives about running. I had come a long way in six years. Yet there was still a lot for me to do. I had been putting off making an entry of my own—for the 2022 Dallas Ultra Marathon.

The difference between a marathon and an ultramarathon is not the distance. It isn't the time, and it isn't the effort. The difference is one of belief: you can believe you can run a marathon, even watch yourself do it, but as soon as you believe yourself capable of running an ultramarathon, you have gotten your foot caught in the first bear trap.

You can only run an ultramarathon once you believe that *no one* can do it and that despite this troubling reality, you are going to do it anyway. That was my takeaway from Oliver's 5K: I believed he could do it, he wasn't sure, and then he did it. In the same way, I wasn't sure if I could run an ultramarathon but, though death or dehydration might stop me, I would make the attempt anyway.

The race was December 11, 2022. The sky over Dallas was cloudy. There was fog all around us. Both impediments seemed inconsequential when compared with the beast that was in front of me. I had run my twentieth marathon only a month prior, in

New York City, but this was different. If I had run fifty marathons in the year up to that point, it still would have seemed like ill preparation for an ultramarathon, defined as anything above either 26.2 miles or 42K (depending on who you ask).

That day, the race stretched fifty kilometers in front of me. I felt prepared to run, but not for *this*. Dressed in my Tracksmith all-black No Days Off tights, a white Tracksmith T-shirt, and baby-blue Nike Air Zoom Alphafly NEXT% 1s, I looked around me for something on the faces, like I always did, and found the same community I had always found, although perhaps just a touch more cautious and reserved than at the more standard-size races.

As we took off through the streets of Dallas, I noted that the feeling of the race became more familiar as we were running. I settled into a groove, reminding myself that I *had* run a marathon only four weeks before.

Then something happened: around mile nineteen, all the ultramarathoners took a turn away from the marathoners and half-marathoners. I knew from studying the track beforehand that this turn would equal about five miles, half there and then half back. As I ran this loop, the crowd around me became sparse. It became harder to find faces to check in on, harder to look for inspiration and motivation anywhere other than my own feet, which were by then crying out to me in angry throbs.

Between miles twenty and twenty-one, there were no spectators, and I never saw more than six runners at a time. No claps, no cheers, no words of encouragement: there was only the solitude of the run, as if we had all coincidentally wandered out onto the streets of Dallas for some early-morning training.

Returning to the pack felt wonderful. It also felt wonderful to see the marker for mile twenty-six, until I remembered that the race wouldn't end, that I still had to do what I had just done *again*.

That was when I stopped—to think about Konstantin Stanislavsky.

I could hear him probing me and goading me on, not to run but to think. As I stood near the marathon finish line, miles of road still in front of me, I asked myself the big questions from Stanislavsky; *Who am I? Why am I here? Where am I coming from? Where am I going?*

Many runners report that after running a marathon, they feel more in touch with themselves than they did beforehand. This transformative power is incredible, and yet I realized it was *not* absolute. Standing on the sidelines and watching Oliver battle and overcome the 5K, I felt wise and accomplished, like I had been there, like I had done that. That feeling is nice, but what is it worth? What good is it to feel wise and accomplished if there may be some road you haven't traveled and if that road may be the one that finally trips you up?

You don't need to see any grunting, struggling faces to know that inside yourself, there's something undone, and if you do it, you can go back to the place from *before* you started collecting all that wisdom and all those accomplishments. You feel new again. Like Oliver, you may ask yourself explicitly, *Can I do this? Should I do this? Is it going to be too much for me?*

Once you rediscover that momentary doubt, you can prove it wrong once more. You can show yourself that it wasn't a fluke and that on both roads taken and untaken, you can keep your feet moving.

While I don't know if I answered any of the biggest questions during the 2022 Dallas Ultra Marathon, I do know that I asked them. I asked them sincerely, availing myself to whatever answers decided to present themselves. I sacrificed for the answers and coolly thought, *Now when those answers are ready to present themselves, I'll be ready to see them.*

Chapter 28

Marathon Globetrotter.

Eight hours for work, another two for the gym, an hour to unwind with a book, a half hour to meditate before bed: we live our lives in a lot of different ways, but whichever ways we are living, we are living *in* time. Time is both the cradle and the grave, there with you through all of your greatest moments. Sometimes you have some extra time, and sometimes you don't have enough. As someone who runs marathons, I think about time a lot, both its demands of me and, in turn, my demands of it. I thought about time even more than usual as I was running the course in Tokyo.

It's a push-and-pull relationship that starts long before I ever line up next to all the other runners. It's every second, and every day, that I get to wake up and breathe, all the hours that I get to look forward to—my life in all its glory.

Early mornings when I wake up or midevenings when the air gets just crisp enough that I can call it perfect, I spend some of my time training. Those hours are some of my favorites. There is no pressure to hit a personal best, but only to run as hard as I can, to get the miles in. Training time adds up quickly. Whenever someone says to me, "You were out there running that race for *three hours*?" I have to smile because those three hours were a fraction of the time I had to invest (or got to invest).

That is how I think about time, almost always. I *get* to invest my time in running. It is a blessing I hold close to my heart. While others must slog off to a warehouse or a factory, off to their offices for another double shift, I am out on the trails and sidewalks. Of course, as anyone who knows me can attest, I can achieve a level of industriousness that would impress even the most dedicated craftsmen and artisans. I love my work, love my studies, and the rhythm of an eight-hour day, but as I need it to be, my schedule is flexible. When a race comes up, I can take time off work. I can use my time *as my own*, which is deeply and inimitably freeing. Nothing about my own life, or my own routine, keeps me from this thing that fills my soul.

None of that is to take away from the effort that we as runners put into our sport. On the contrary, we *choose* to spend our time running a marathon.

The privilege of it all is undeniable, though. To have the money to put into running is a privilege as well. These costs, like the time of training, add up. New kicks, every registration, all the travel expenses, special meals to maintain my body: the bills would cause many people to blush. Yet I would spend that money no other way, just as I would spend that time no other way. It is a beautiful experience, mile after mile, and when my toes are tapping against the ground and the cold wind is all the respite my lungs need, I know that I have made the right decisions, from registration to training to race day itself.

Race day itself: before we get there, let's go back a few legs.

Proust, who wrote *À la Recherche du Temps Perdu* (*In Search of Lost Time* or, originally, *A Remembrance of Things Past*), said, "Time passes, and little by little everything that we have spoken in falsehood becomes true." Think about the privilege that change and reflection represent: For the person who spends a lifetime sewing at a table or ringing up other people's snacks on a cash register, there is very little time to stop and change. There is little time for perspective, which running gifts to me in droves. I am forever changing, constantly observing my own mind while the mile markers are a blur on the side of the road and old falsehoods become truths.

Old convictions become follies I've outgrown.

I have descended into the pits of my own memories and beliefs, tearing them apart, picking at them until some light started to show through on the other side. None of that would have been possible without running, without the peace of time running affords me.

Again, it's not merely the time on the course.

It's the time traveling too. For the Tokyo Marathon in 2023, there was plenty of that. I marveled, in the weeks and months leading up to the race, that I would get *so much* time before the morning-of. I would spend several multiples more time getting to the race than I would spend running it.

My journey had begun in New York City: that was the first of the Abbott World Marathon Majors I had run. A taxi, a ferry, and a bus. None of the travel time was, as every New Yorker could guess, anything like Waze would have suggested. There were delays, red lights that ran longer than it seemed they should have, and at every delay, there was more time to ponder the day ahead. Later in Boston, the time was on Amtrak, through the tunnel that the locals will always call the Big Dig, mockery in their *R*-less accents. Chicago had required me to take a plane, as had Berlin and London. Five races and many, many hours of travel time.

Tokyo, of course, was the longest trip of all. In total, I spent fourteen hours getting from New York City to there; a ninety-minute layover; ten hours to Sydney, Australia, for a brief sojourn; and ten hours back to Tokyo. All that time, one can't help but feel like the quest ahead is worth taking, like there is something to find out there in all those ticking minutes and their refusal to slow down, speed up, or stop.

The time becomes a keeper of itself in that sense. While it's passing, I am passing with it. That is time's other characteristic, the one that we usually talk about in whispers. It is wearing each of us away. The sands of time are literal for our bodies, just like they are literal for the mountains that the waves beat down into oblivion.

Sometimes, time is rougher than that. The wrong moment can, without any warning, take everything away.

When I am out on one of the courses, I think about the people who have been unlucky in that regard. I think about their families, what it would mean for them to see their loved ones running too. As I prepared for the Tokyo Marathon in 2019, I raised money for charity because of the feeling of *goodness* that all the other races had instilled in me. It turned out that their rules were a little different from what I was used to, as they would only accept the first few thousand runners to hit their target.

Flash-forward to 2020: I raised my money earlier this time, for the Tokyo Toy Museum, and submitted my application to compete in the 2020 Tokyo Marathon. The date was set: March 1, 2020. Of course, that race didn't happen. Japan closed its borders, and I didn't run a single marathon that year. Because I missed an email, I didn't get to run the 2021 New York City Marathon either. I returned to the majors in 2022, in New York City for my twentieth marathon and in Dallas for my twenty-first.

By the time I was back on my six-star journey, three years had passed. I was five out of six—one race away from the coveted, shimmering six-star medal. It would be one of the most shining accomplishments in my life as a runner.

I was *ready.*

Then, just as the pandemic had once before, life and time came toppling down on me. I was ten days out from the Tokyo Marathon, in Arkansas for a writing residency, far from home. All my thoughts were halfway across the Pacific when I took a tumble down a stairway. The pain was immediate and haunting. It mocked me while I lay there on the ground.

As soon as I could, I visited a doctor in Bentonville. His news was bleak. "It's definitely broken," he said to me as all those years and all that sweat, every grain of time, all slipped through my fingers.

I flew back to New York City, storing my crutches in the overhead bin. Since the doctor in Bentonville hadn't done an X-ray, I held on to some hope. That seemed like my right if a stairway was going to rip this dream away from me. The six stars' light was dimming, and I didn't intend to let them go all the way out, not without putting up a fight.

In New York City, the second opinion was less severe, but only slightly. The doctor said, "It's most likely not broken, but in extremely bad shape."

"Let's do an X-ray," I said.

"Isn't the pain . . . ?"

"Excruciating," I said. "Some of the worst of my life, but not so bad as the other day. I'm running the Tokyo Marathon in eight days, though."

"No, you're not," the doctor said. "Not in this condition."

I insisted on the X-ray, which I could tell the doctor *hated*. However, his frustration and shock morphed into surprise and confusion when he read the X-ray.

"It's not broken," he said. "Not only that, but it's only a very slight sprain."

It was the best thing he could have said to me. Although he seemed not to appreciate the mischievous grin that crept up on my face, knowing that no sprain would keep me from Tokyo, the moments were mine again. I had reclaimed my time from the couch and the cats that had threatened to confine me.

I would cross that finish line and earn my sixth star.

After I arrived in Tokyo, I spent another ten hours flying to Sydney, where I saw *La Bohéme* performed at the Sydney Opera House. I sat front and center, close enough to reach out and tug the conductor's jacket (which I opted not to do).

On race day, I marveled at how organized the Japanese event managers were. I felt like an expert on the matter, having run the first five of six. It was a feat of engineering: All the runners who had registered for 2020, 2021, and 2022 lined up there next to me. We had all missed this moment once before, and we weren't going to miss it again. According to Guinness World Records, that day featured more six-star finishers than any other time in history—three thousand, almost half of the all-time total, because of the delays that we had faced, because of the gumption and resilience that had carried us across oceans and through painful nights training and even more painful nights wondering if the training would all be for naught, hoping that the world would start spinning again and our time would be our own once more.

At the nineteenth mile, there was a pang in my ankle. My mind went back to Bentonville, to CityMD, to every trail I had paced, to the clock on my phone and the minutes and hours that it beat away.

My mind went to Proust. I was searching for lost time of my own, for the years that I hadn't run and the years I had gotten to run, for five stars under my belt and a sixth only seven miles away. It wouldn't stop me: That ankle could have snapped in two and I would have crawled the last 10K and more. It meant too much—everything—and as I crossed the finish line, I hardly noticed any pain at all.

My friend Andrew and I had met five years prior, at the Abbott World Marathon Majors event in Berlin. He earned his sixth star in Tokyo that day as well. We celebrated that night with sushi and sake. It was everything that we could have hoped it would be, to live life fully in a faraway land like that and to know that despite the slings and arrows of 2020, 2021, and 2022, we had become six-star runners.

Lil Wayne rapped, "If we could buy time, every store would sell it." As it is, we can't do that. We can't buy or sell time. We can invest it, we can use it up, we can throw it away, and we can cherish it. We can use it for something that we deem fit and if there's enough of it left over at the end of a day. All those days, there was something left over for me, enough moments for me to schedule a short run or even a long run, so much time on a weekend that I could spend it in the Big Apple, or among the skyscrapers of Berlin, in Chicago and Boston and London, in Tokyo, where five stars had become six—and time took a pause as my feet came to a stop and the joy of the medal was mine. The joy of running has given me so much and has offered a great deal of perspective on race, racing, fitness, justice, and time.

Like the martial artist who finally earns his coveted black belt, only to learn that is where the true learning and training begins; I, too, realized that after earning my sixth star in Tokyo, my true learning and training had only just begun. There are more races to run and many more personal and life lessons to master—time well spent.

Printed in the USA
CPSIA information can be obtained
at www.ICGtesting.com
LVHW051826301023
762208LV00036B/435/J